STEP-BY-STEP
HAIRSTYLES
85 SALON LOOKS TO CREATE

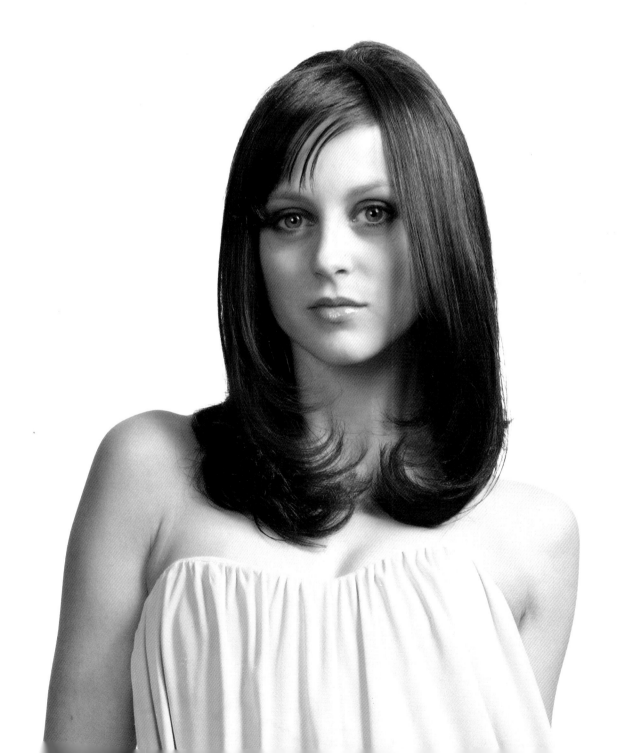

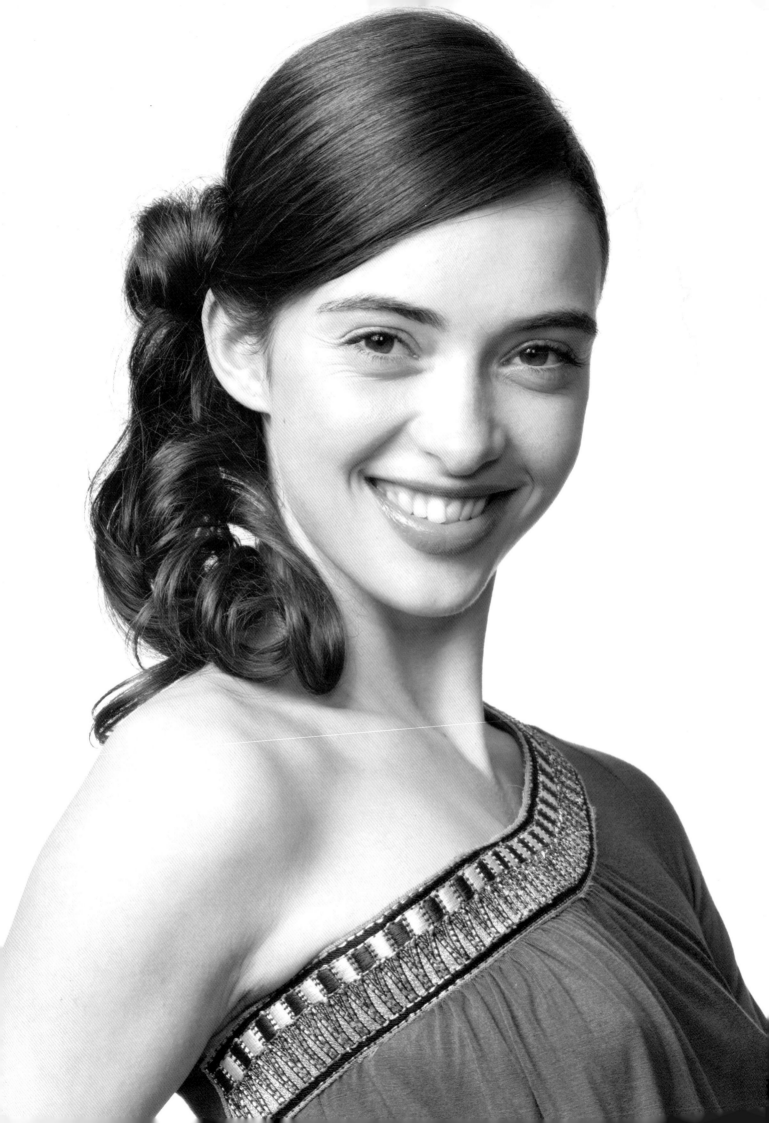

STEP-BY-STEP
HAIRSTYLES
85 SALON LOOKS TO CREATE

A comprehensive practical guide to styling your hair for stunning results, with more than 85 complete looks shown in 500 how-to photographs

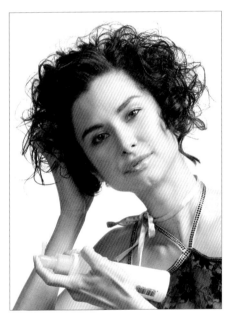
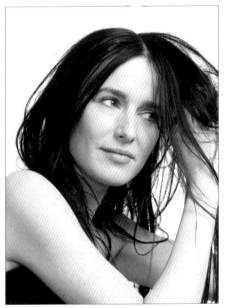
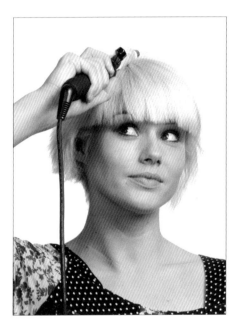

Nicky Pope

Photography by David Goldman

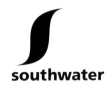

southwater

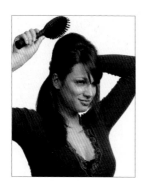 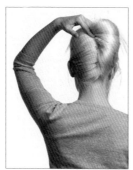 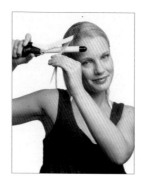 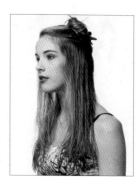 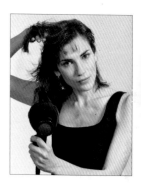

This edition is published by Southwater, an imprint of Anness Publishing Ltd, Blaby Road, Wigston, Leicestershire LE18 4SE; info@anness.com

www.southwaterbooks.com;
www.annesspublishing.com

If you like the images in this book and would like to investigate using them for publishing, promotions or advertising, please visit our website www.practicalpictures.com for more information.

Publisher: Joanna Lorenz
Senior Editor: Lucy Doncaster
Project Editor: Dan Hurst
Designer: Simon Daley
Jacket Designer: Lisa Tai
Illustrator: Vanessa Card
Production Controller: Bessie Bai

© Anness Publishing Ltd 2012

A CIP catalogue record for this book is available from the British Library.

Previously published as part of a larger volume, *The Professional's Illustrated Guide to Haircare & Hairstyles*.

PUBLISHER'S NOTE
Although the advice and information in this book are believed to be accurate and true at the time of going to press, neither the authors nor the publisher can accept any legal responsiblity or liability for any errors or omissions that may have been made nor for any inaccuracies nor for any loss, harm or injury that comes about from following instructions or advice in this book. All electrical equipment should be used with caution and should never be left unattended.

Bracketed terms are intended for American readers.

AUTHOR'S NOTE
Special thanks for their encouragement and help to Louise Wood and Susan Pope for being my second eyes, and to Tim Frisby for getting me started. I'm grateful to Lucy Doncaster for being unflappable, patient and very good at what she does.

ETHICAL TRADING POLICY
At Anness Publishing we believe that business should be conducted in an ethical and ecologically sustainable way, with respect for the environment and a proper regard to the replacement of the natural resources we employ.

As a publisher, we use a lot of wood pulp in high-quality paper for printing, and that wood commonly comes from spruce trees. We are therefore currently growing more than 750,000 trees in three Scottish forest plantations: Berrymoss (130 hectares/320 acres), West Touxhill (125 hectares/305 acres) and Deveron Forest (75 hectares/185 acres). The forests we manage contain more than 3.5 times the number of trees employed each year in making paper for the books we manufacture.

Because of this ongoing ecological investment programme, you, as our customer, can have the pleasure and reassurance of knowing that a tree is being cultivated on your behalf to naturally replace the materials used to make the book you are holding.

Our forestry programme is run in accordance with the UK Woodland Assurance Scheme (UKWAS) and will be certified by the internationally recognized Forest Stewardship Council (FSC). The FSC is a non-government organization dedicated to promoting responsible management of the world's forests. Certification ensures forests are managed in an environmentally sustainable and socially responsible way. For further information about this scheme, go to www.annesspublishing.com/trees

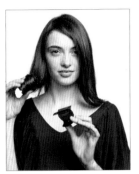
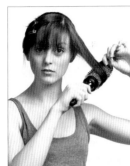
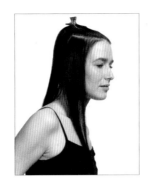
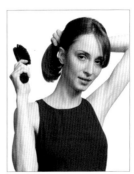
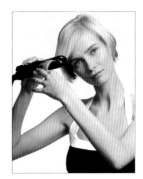

CONTENTS

Introduction **6**

STYLING TOOLS AND PRODUCTS 8

Styling tools **10** ▪ Heated appliances **14** ▪ Styling products **16** ▪ Basic styling techniques **18**

EVERYDAY STYLING TECHNIQUES 20

Blow-drying shorter hair for a smooth finish **22** ▪ Blow-drying shorter hair smooth with kicked-out ends **23** ▪ Blow-drying shorter hair for a chic, grown-up look **24** ▪ Blow-drying shorter hair for a sleek, shiny finish **25** ▪ Blow-drying the perfect long bob **26** ▪ Blow-drying shorter hair for a soft, relaxed look **28** ▪ Blow-drying shorter hair for a multi-texture effect **30** ▪ Blow-drying shorter hair for a textured finish **32** ▪ Blow-drying to add contrast to a shorter textured style **33** ▪ Blow-drying to add volume and choppy texture to shorter hair **34** ▪ Blow-drying mid-length hair for all-over texture **35** ▪ Blow-drying fringed mid-length hair for a textured finish **36** ▪ Blow-drying mid-length or longer hair for a loose finish **37** ▪ Blow-drying mid-length or longer hair to curl under **38** ▪ Blow-drying mid-length or longer hair for a bedhead finish **39** ▪ Blow-drying longer hair for a smooth finish **40** ▪ Blow-drying longer hair for volume and movement **42** ▪ Blow-drying curly hair for a soft, smooth look **44** ▪ Blow-drying to add emphasis to a deep, wide fringe **46** ▪ Tonging shorter hair for texture **47** ▪ Using tongs for different curled effects **48** ▪ Using tongs to create random spiral curls **50** ▪ Using tongs to create all-over curl **51** ▪ Using irons to create striking blades in shorter hair **52** ▪ Using irons to create movement in shorter hair **54** ▪ Using irons to create flicks in layered or graduated hair **55** ▪ Using irons to straighten hair for a super-sleek look **56** ▪ Using irons to create movement in longer hair **58** ▪ Crimping loose hair for all-over texture **60** ▪ Crimping dressed hair for partial texture **62** ▪ Crimping loose hair for a random texture effect **63** ▪ Setting hair on heated rollers **64** ▪ Setting hair on self-gripping rollers **65** ▪ Using bendable rods to create an even curl **66** ▪ Using pin curls to create a gentle, tumbling curl **68** ▪ Using barrel curls to create volume and soft curl **69** ▪ Using plaits to create a gentle wave **70** ▪ Using multi-plaits to create a stronger wave **71** ▪ Forming a Marcel wave for a retro look **72** ▪ Using your fingers to shape shorter hair **73** ▪ Using gel to create a smooth, wet look on shorter hair **74** ▪ Using gel to create spikes on shorter hair **75** ▪ Using mousse to create a bedhead finish on longer hair **76** ▪ Fitting and wearing a wig with a natural hair fringe **77** ▪ Fitting and wearing a whole-head wig **78** ▪ Fitting and wearing a hair weft **80** ▪ Fitting and wearing a false fringe **81** ▪ Fitting and wearing a false ponytail **82** ▪ A range of fringe finishes for different effects **84** ▪ Creating a rolling ponytail on mid-length or longer hair **86** ▪ Placing ponytails for different effects **88** ▪ Creating a perfect plaited ponytail **90** ▪ Creating a perfect ballerina bun **92** ▪ Creating a perfect French roll **94** ▪ Creating a perfect woven bun **96** ▪ Creating a perfect French pleat **98** ▪ Creating a sweet asymmetric back-do **100** ▪ Creating a textured twist up-do on longer hair **102**

SPECIAL OCCASIONS 104

Creating a sleek, elegant finish on shorter hair **106** ▪ Creating a glamorous pin-up on shorter curly hair **107** ▪ Creating a quick, chic party look on shorter hair **108** ▪ Creating a quick party look on mid-length hair **110** ▪ Creating a quick party look on curly hair **112** ▪ Creating a perfect wave set **114** ▪ Creating sumptuous curls on straight hair **116** ▪ Creating sophisticated ponytails for special events **118** ▪ Creating a slick offset ballerina bun **120** ▪ Creating a perfect classic chignon **122** ▪ Creating a pin-up on mid-length hair **124** ▪ Creating a twist back-do on mid-length hair **126** ▪ Creating a twist up-do on longer hair **127** ▪ Creating a mussed-up back-do on mid-length hair **128** ▪ Creating a glamorous back-do **130** ▪ Creating a back-do with extra height **132** ▪ Creating an elegant top roll up-do **134** ▪ Creating an up-do with a front roll detail **136** ▪ Creating a chic, tonged tumbling up-do **138** ▪ Creating an up-do on curly hair **140** ▪ Creating an up-do on crimped hair **142** ▪ Creating a loose wedding style **144** ▪ Creating a stylish wedding back-do **145** ▪ Creating a contemporary wedding back-do **146** ▪ Creating a classic wedding back-do **147** ▪ Creating a romantic wedding pin-up **148** ▪ Creating a chic wedding up-do **149** ▪ Wearing a hat **150** ▪ Formal hats **152** ▪ Informal hats **153** ▪ Choosing accessories **154** ▪ Flowers **155** ▪ Hairgrips and hair slides **156** ▪ Bows and ribbons **157**

Index **158**
Acknowledgements **160**

Introduction

How you wear your hair and the way it makes you look and feel is incredibly important. Whether hair is groomed, worn loose and casual, or even remains unkempt, do remember that its look, colour, texture and style is all part of your individuality.

Although genetic factors determine the type, natural colour and texture of your hair, the rest is down to you. The way you live your life, your state of health and your haircare regime will impact on the overall appearance of your hair and its capacity to shine, move and look vital. Beyond that the many styling options available to you mean that it is possible to reinvent your look on a daily basis, from dramatic cut and colour changes through to simple and temporary styling techniques.

For many centuries women all over the world have been changing the colour of their hair, originally using dyes made from natural sources such as henna and, in more modern times, from chemical colourants, although natural dyes are still very popular and widely available.

The desire to curl or wave straight hair or smooth out natural curls is also pervasive in most cultures, and as new techniques and tools develop, the power of a hairstyle to entirely change a person's look becomes ever more apparent – it's almost a magical way to reinvent an identity.

It's no surprise, then, that so many women spend time and energy in getting their hair to look a certain way, and stay like that. From hours in the bathroom, washing, fixing and styling hair, to countless trips to the salon for cut, colour and waving services, it seems that hair and hairdressing is bigger business than ever. But with so much advice available, so many products and such a choice of hairstyling tools and equipment spilling off shelves in the shops, it's not quite so easy to figure out what to do for the best! How will you know what style is right for you? How should you care for your hair and make sure every day is a good hair day?

The answers lie in understanding your hair and learning to manage it well, and this beautiful book tells everything you will ever need to know about your hair, from basic care to styling and dressing it yourself so that you can be confident that your hair looks fantastic each time you step out of the door.

The book opens with a chapter on styling tools and products that comprehensively explains what to use and when, together with valuable information on styling and finishing products. This section looks at essential styling tools, such as the range of hairbrushes available, and explains the practical uses of each one. It also offers invaluable information on pins and

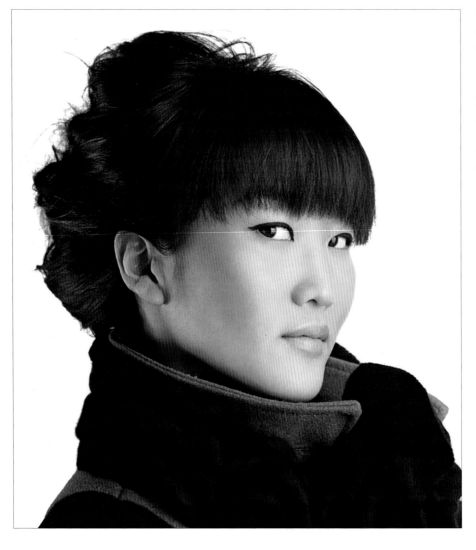

Left *Regard your hair as an asset. Shiny, healthy hair dressed to suit your individual look is an important part of your personal style.*

clips, rollers, shapers and rods and demonstrates how to implement them into your styling and haircare regime. The section on heated appliances looks in detail at hairdryers, straightening and crimping irons, curling tongs, hot brushes, heated rollers and hot sticks. The use of each tool is clearly explained, and handy styling tips ensure that the reader is fully prepared to embark upon styling their hair in new and exciting ways. Forget indecision and feelings of panic as you gain an insight into superb styling for every occasion.

Having laid the foundations, the book continues by exploring ways of dressing hair, with pages of clearly illustrated step-by-step explanations for a range of styling techniques, from basic blow-dries to straightening, curling and setting hair in a variety of ways, using rods, bendies, curlers and pins. You can practise affixing temporary hair, too, including ponytails, flashes of colour and even full wigs.

There are more than 85 projects you can undertake at home, and each sequence is illustrated with easy-to-follow step-by-step photographs. The styles range from easy ideas for casual daywear through to slick work styles and then on to party nights and special occasions, from glamorous red carpet dos to romantic and elegant wedding-day styles.

Having revealed the secrets of how to achieve perfect hairstyles, it makes sense to consider how best to wear a hat to suit your hair, and we show you how to

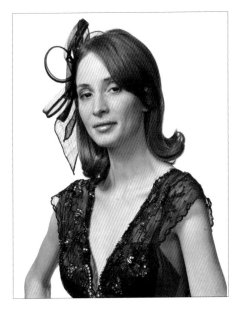

Above Learn how to wear accessories, hats and ornaments in a way that balances your face shape and works with your dress style.

select something right for any occasion, as well as how to make your own headpiece. Accessories such as flowers, bows and clips, scarves and headbands are another great way to add a finishing touch to a hairstyle and we share ideas on what to wear and how to fix it to your hair for a stylish and truly individual finish.

Hair is a good indicator of your health, personality and mood, so enjoy its potential and bring out the best in yourself. Learn to love your hair and wear it with style.

Below An elegant hair ornament adds glamour and individuality to any hairstyle, and can transform a look from day to evening.

Left Practise good haircare and follow a styling routine to keep your hair looking in great condition at all times.

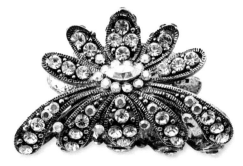

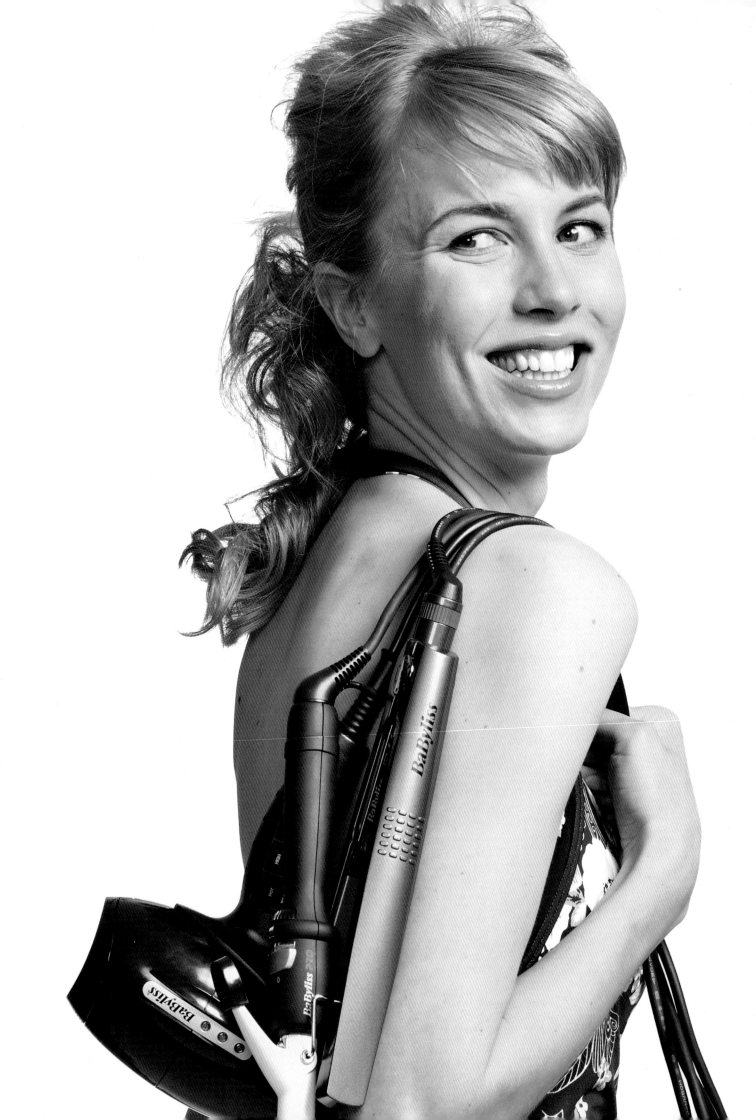

Styling tools and products

Beautiful, shining hair can and should make you look
and feel great. It is a versatile fashion accessory, and
you can change its colour, texture, shape and length
to suit your mood and personal style. There is a huge
range of hairbrushes, combs, accessories, tools, and
heated styling appliances available to help you
achieve these changes, and a wide variety of
products to ensure that your hair is always looking its
best. This chapter reveals what these tools and
products are, how they are used and offers useful
advice on how to adapt their uses to suit your style.

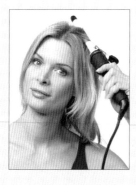 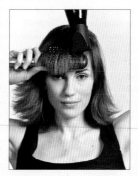 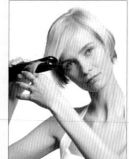

Styling tools

The right tools not only make hairstyling easier, but mean you can be more versatile, too. Hairbrushes, combs and pins are the basic tools of styling and today the choice is enormous. The following is a quick guide to help you choose what is most suitable.

Hairbrushes

A device for detangling, smoothing and shaping hair, a hairbrush comprises bristles (sometimes termed quills or pins), which may be made from natural hog bristle, plastic, nylon or wire, and which are embedded in a wooden, plastic or moulded rubber base and set in tufts or rows. Arranging bristles like this allows loose hair to collect in the grooves without interfering with the action of the bristles moving through your hair. The spacing of the tufts plays an important role – generally, the wider the spacing between the rows of bristles the easier the hairbrush will flow.

The purpose of brushing is to remove tangles and knots and generally smooth the hair. The action of brushing from the roots to the ends removes dead skin cells and dirt, and encourages the cuticles to lie flat, thus reflecting the light. Brushing also stimulates the blood supply to the hair follicles, promoting healthy growth.

Natural bristles are made of natural keratin (the same material as hair) and therefore create less friction and wear on the hair. They are good for grooming and polishing, and help to combat static on flyaway hair. However, they will not easily penetrate wet or thick hair and you must

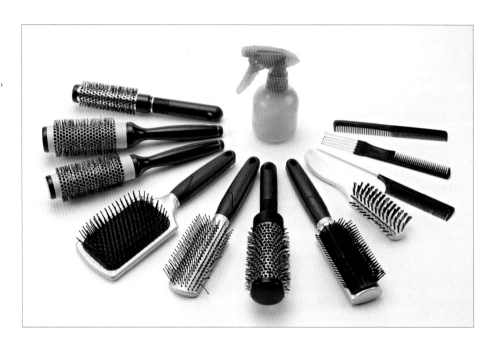

Above *There are many types of brushes to use depending on your choice of style and hair type. Keep several so you are prepared at all times.*

use a softer bristle brush for fine or thinning hair. In addition, the sharp ends can scratch the scalp.

Plastic, nylon or wire bristles are easily cleaned and usually heat-resistant, so they can be used when you are blow-drying, but they may distort if subjected to extreme heat.

▪ Flat or half-round brushes

Ideal for all aspects of wet or dry styling and blow-drying, flat or half-round brushes are good all-round tools but are not precise enough for serious styling, which is where round brushes come in.

Closely set bristles on a flat brush are useful for creating smooth, straight styles where hair isn't long enough to lie easily on the brush. Widely-spaced, thick bristles are ideal for smoothing straight hair which is longer. You can

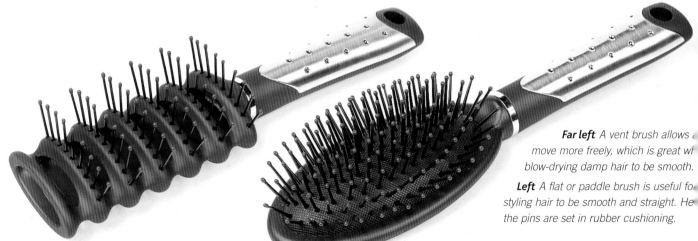

Far left *A vent brush allows a move more freely, which is great wh blow-drying damp hair to be smooth.*

Left *A flat or paddle brush is useful fo styling hair to be smooth and straight. He the pins are set in rubber cushioning.*

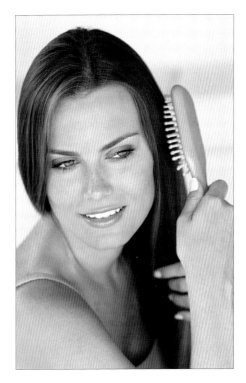

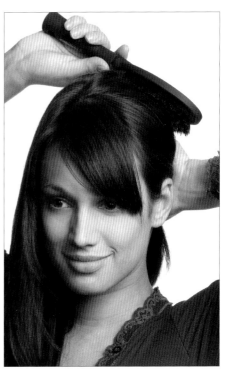

Far right Use a softer bristle if your hair is prone to breakages or split ends and don't brush too vigorously or you will stress the hair further.

Right A flat-backed brush smoothes hair and is easily drawn through longer styles, making it lie flat.

also use a flat brush to create flicks and movement, drawing the brush through the hair, then turning it out as you reach the ends of the hair.

- **Paddle brushes**

Broad, flat, paddle brushes are great for blow-drying wavy hair to be straight, as well as achieving a poker-straight finish on long hair. Rubber cushioning on the paddle can ensure an extra-smooth, static-free finish.

- **Pneumatic brushes**

These popular brushes have a domed, air-cushioned rubber base with bristles set in tufts. They can be plastic, natural bristle or both and are great for smoothing all types of hair and countering static electricity. The nylon bristles offer more grip for detangling while the natural ones are super-smoothing and perfect for thinner hair.

- **Vent brushes**

Usually made from plastic, vent brushes have vented, hollow centres that allow the airflow from the dryer to pass through them. Special bristle or pin patterns are designed to lift and disentangle even wet hair. Vents and tunnel brush heads enable the air to circulate freely through both the brush and the hair so the hair dries faster.

- **Circular or radial brushes**

These brushes come in a variety of sizes and are circular or semi-circular in shape.

Close-set bristles tend to grip the hair more tightly, while widely set bristles will control the air more easily and help remove tangles.

The development of metal or ceramic barrels has been popular as this helps the brush retain heat and better shape the hair (like a roller) when used with a hairdryer. Use these brushes to:

- Tame and control naturally curly, permed and wavy hair.
- Smooth hair during blow-drying; you can draw them through the hair and achieve a smooth finish.
- Create wave or curl when blow-drying – wrapping hair round them and using like a large roller. Leave the brush in the hair as it cools to promote better curl retention.

- Achieve root lift by using the brush to lift the hair away from your head as you blow-dry. The diameter of the barrel of the brush determines the resulting volume and movement: a large diameter creates a soft curl; a smaller one creates a tighter curl. Remember when choosing a radial brush with a large diameter that your hair must be long enough to wrap around it, so don't buy a large brush if you only have short hair.

- **Dressing-out brushes**

These are narrow brushes with only a few rows of bristles set into the head, and they have a tail. They are designed for back-brushing hair at the roots when creating volume and lift, particularly when dressing hair.

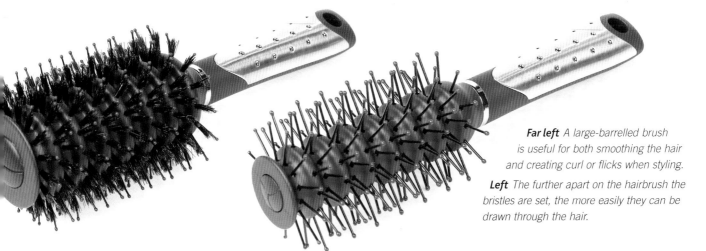

Far left A large-barrelled brush is useful for both smoothing the hair and creating curl or flicks when styling.

Left The further apart on the hairbrush the bristles are set, the more easily they can be drawn through the hair.

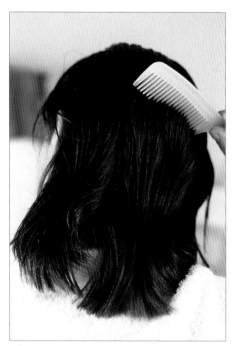

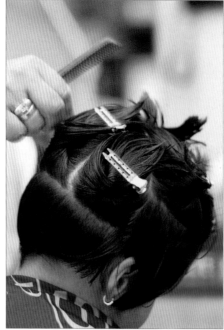

Above Use a comb rather than a brush on damp hair, since it stretches and breaks more easily than dry hair and requires gentle care.

Above Flat sectioning clips are great for sectioning hair and for using to hold pin curls in place while hair dries.

Clockwise, from top left Small sectioning clips; snap clips; open-ended fine hair pins and hairgrips (bobby pins).

Combs

Choose good-quality combs with saw-cut teeth. This means that each individual tooth is cut into the comb, so there are no sharp edges. Avoid cheap plastic combs that are made in a mould and so form lines down the centre of every tooth, and replace combs that have damaged teeth. They are sharp, and scrape away the cuticle layers of the hair, causing damage.

- **Wide-toothed combs** are used for disentangling and combing conditioner through the hair.
- **Fine-tail combs** are for styling and sectioning hair. They are the only way to create the perfect parting!
- **Afro combs** are for curly hair as they don't snag as easily.

Pins and clips

Endlessly versatile and cheap, there are several different types to choose from:
- **Open-ended and fine hair pins** are used for securing hair, especially for up-dos such as into chignons. They are quite delicate and prone to bend out of shape, so they should only be used to secure small amounts of hair. These pins are easily concealed, especially if you use a matching colour. They are sometimes used to secure pin curls during setting, rather than heavier clips, which can leave a mark.
- **Twisted pins** are similar to open-ended pins but are fashioned like a screw and are used to secure French pleats (rolls) and chignons.

- **Hairgrips (bobby pins)** are closed hairgrips that lie flat to the head. Prise them apart to slide into the hair and push in as far as possible to help conceal them in the hair. They come in a variety of colours, so choose hairgrips to suit.
- **Sectioning clips** are clips with a double prong that snaps shut, and are longer in length than other clips. They are most often used for holding hair out of the way while working on another section, or for securing pin curls.
- **Snap clips** are stronger and hold more hair than hairgrips but are more difficult to conceal. They snap open so you can pass hair between the outer rim and the inner prong, then snap shut. They are available in different colours.

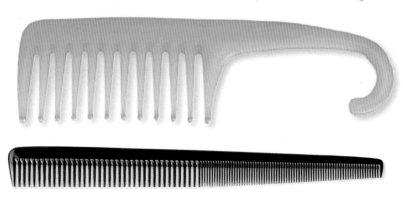

Far top left A wide-toothed saw-cut comb is a necessity for any hair care regime, especially for detangling wet hair, which can be fragile.

Far bottom left Fine combs are an essential tool for getting a professional-looking finish when styling hair.

Left Afro combs should be used for very curly hair, for lifting the root area without snagging and tearing hair.

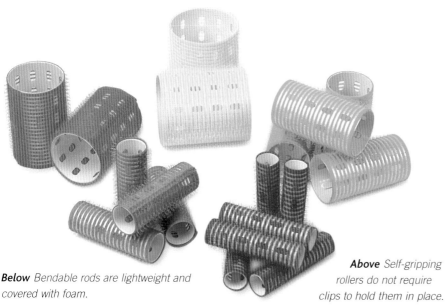

Above Self-gripping rollers do not require clips to hold them in place.

Shapers or rods

Producing soft, bouncy curls, shapers or rods are extremely useful pieces of equipment. They were inspired by the principle of rag-rolling hair. Soft 'twist tie' ones are made from pliable rubber, plastic or cotton fabric and provide one of the more natural ways to curl hair. In the centre of each shaper is a tempered wire, which enables it to be bent into shape. The technique is gentle enough for fragile permed or tinted hair.

To use, section clean, dry hair and pull to a firm tension, 'trapping' the end in a shaper that you have previously doubled over. Roll down to the roots of the hair and fold over to secure. Leave in for 30–60 minutes without heat, or for 10–15 minutes if you apply heat. If you twist the hair before curling you will achieve a more voluminous style.

Below left Heated rollers are placed in the hair and held in place with bespoke clips, then left to cool.

Below Up-dos often require hair to be set on rollers or curled on tongs to add movement and guts to give shape and volume to the hair.

Below Bendable rods are lightweight and covered with foam.

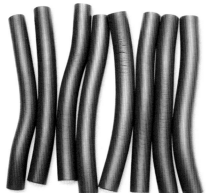

Rollers

Invaluable for creating wave and curl, rollers vary in diameter, length and the material from which they are made:
- **Smooth rollers** do not have spikes or brushes and will give the sleekest finish, but are more difficult to put in.
- **Brush rollers** are more popular, especially the self-holding variety that do not require pins or clips.

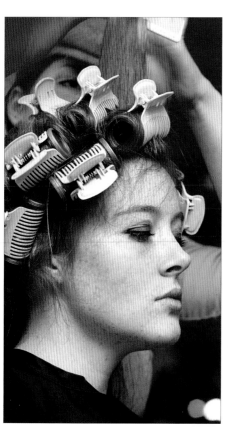

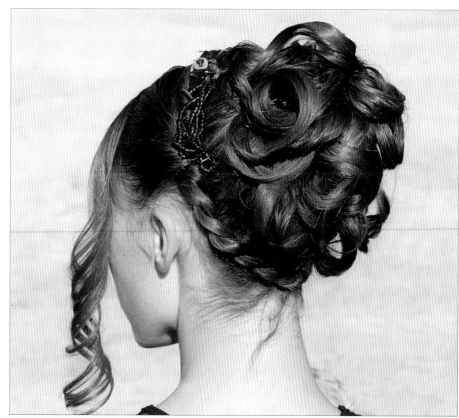

Heated appliances

A wide range of gadgets is available for styling your hair quickly and easily, and continuing technological developments mean there are always new and improved products to try. Here's a guide to the main categories and what they do.

Modern technology

Electrical styling tools make great use of a range of different technologies and materials, including:

• **Ionic technology** utilizes negative ions to remove moisture from the hair more quickly. The negative ions break water molecules into smaller particles, which then evaporate faster, cutting drying time. They also help to tighten the hair cuticle, making hair softer and more shiny and reducing frizz.

• **Ceramic heat elements** are great for spreading heat more evenly so you can style hair using a milder heat. Arguably, ceramic plates on irons or tongs are smoother and kinder to the hair than other materials.

• **Far infrared** technology is a new understanding of how to use far infrared rays to help to shorten drying time and reduce damage to the hair from direct heat.

• **Tourmaline** is a mineral compound (similar to ceramic) that emits negative ions and infrared. When incorporated into a dryer design, it can help seal in moisture and dry hair faster. In styling tools, some believe that it produces a smoother, more shiny finish to the hair. Tourmaline and ceramic substances are often combined in the same piece of equipment.

Hairdryers

Used for drying wet hair, hairdryers can also make your hair super-smooth, straight or wavy, add lift and volume.

Narrow nozzles can be fitted on to the end of the hairdryer cylinder and they direct air-flow for precision drying. This is especially useful when smoothing hair. Alternatively, diffuser attachments spread the airflow over the hair to dry it more slowly, with the intention of retaining texture, especially in curly hair, which can become frizzy if you use a standard nozzle.

Travel dryers are ideal for taking on trips and are usually miniature versions of standard dryers. Check you have one with dual voltage. When buying a standard dryer, look out for the following key features:

• A motor of at least 1500 watts (this refers to the power of the motor and how fast it works, decreasing the drying time).

• High- and low-power settings.

• Temperature options and a cool-shot button (for a blast of cold air when you need it).

• Ionic technology, which represents a great step forward in the performance and improved drying times of hairdryers available today.

Drying tips

• Always point the dryer so the air flows down the hair shaft to smooth the cuticle and encourage shine.

• Take care not to hold the dryer too near the scalp; it can cause burns.

• When you have finished blow-drying, allow the hair to cool thoroughly, then check that the hair is completely dry. Warm hair often gives the illusion of dryness while it is, in fact, still damp.

• Never use a dryer without its filter in place – hair can easily be drawn into the machine where it will get caught.

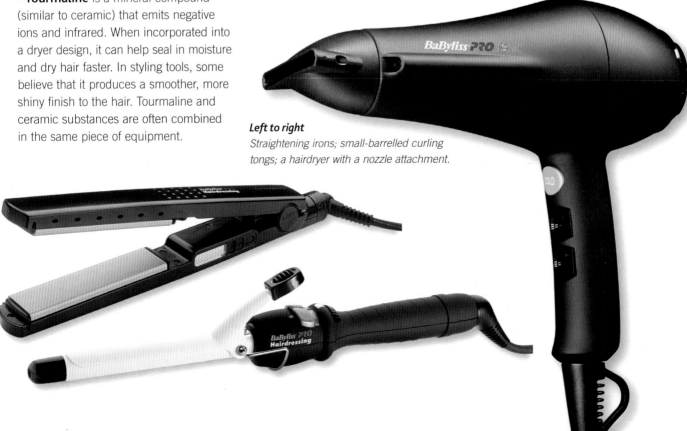

Left to right
Straightening irons; small-barrelled curling tongs; a hairdryer with a nozzle attachment.

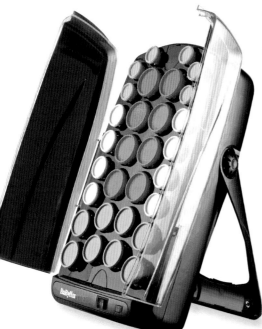

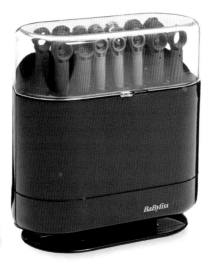

Left Heated rollers come in many formats, including these upright display rollers.
Below Hot sticks are bendable rods that work like small-diameter rollers.

New developments include ribbed rubber surfaces, which are designed to be kinder to the hair; curved barrel shapes that follow the form of the head, and clip fasteners.

Hot sticks
Similar to bendable rods or shapers, these are pliable heated sticks that are self-holding (by bending the ends), so no clips are required. Available in ceramic and non-ceramic versions, you place them in the hair when they are hot, twist to fix in place and leave to cool for small, tight curl results.

Styling tips
- Heat-drying encourages static, causing hair to fly away. You can reduce this by smoothing down your hair with your hand.
- With the exception of hairdryers, always use heated electrical styling tools on dry, not wet, hair.
- If you are curling tight up to the roots, try placing a comb between the tongs and the scalp so the comb forms a barrier against the heat and helps to prevent scalp burns.
- Leave tonged curls to cool completely before styling.

Straightening irons
Sometimes called flat irons, straightening irons have two heated flat plates which are clamped over a section of hair and slowly drawn to the ends, literally ironing hair as flat and smooth as possible. They can be used to press curly hair, and help tame frizzy hair.

Today, irons are designed with heat controls, either as a digital display unit on the cord or on the iron itself. There is a choice of plate sizes and widths suitable for hair of any length, and they are also available with round-backs, which make it possible to wave the hair (by wrapping sections of hair round the iron before drawing them between the heated plates).

Developments in ionic technology and the use of ceramic plates have improved heat distribution and performance considerably, making irons one of the most versatile styling tools available.

Crimping irons
These irons consist of two ridged, metal plates that are corrugated to produce uniform patterned crimps in straight lines in the hair. Some crimpers have reversible or dual-effect styling plates to give different finishes. Use for special looks or to increase volume. Use only on dry hair that has been spritzed with heat-protective spray to prevent scorching.

Curling tongs
Tongs consist of a barrel, or prong, and a grooved 'depressor' which fits against the barrel and works on a spring action so that hair can be wrapped round the barrel and clamped to hold.

The diameter of the barrel and the size of tong is varied according to the size of curl you want to create and the length of your hair. Use tongs only on dry hair that has been spritzed with heat-protective spray to avoid scorching the hair.

Hot brushes
Looking similar to a curling tong but without the depressor, hot brushes have bristles to grab the hair when wrapping sections to form curls. Hot brushes also come in varying diameters for creating curls of different sizes. Arguably they are best for short to medium length hair and particularly for lifting at the roots.

Heated rollers
Available in sets, heated rollers normally comprise a selection of around 20 small, medium and large rollers, with colour-coded clips of different sizes to match. The early models came with spikes, which many women prefer because they have a good grip, but smooth rollers (held in place with bespoke clips) arguably give a better finish.

Styling products

Styling and finishing products are designed to help make hair more manageable during the drying and styling process and retain the style longer. They also have conditioning actions to help compensate for the damage done during heat styling.

The combination of practice and the right styling product will enable you to achieve a salon finish at home, so it is worth checking out what does what and how each can help your particular hair type. Many will also be available in a variety of hold strengths, often called hold-factor, ranging from light to extra-firm.

Style it

- **Blow-dry lotions, styling crèmes and sprays** are usually a single-application product that is distributed evenly all over the hair using fingers. They add guts and hold when drying the hair to help maintain the new style. They are similar to leave-in conditioner as they help to limit damage to the hair during styling.
- **Mousse** is the most versatile styling product. It comes as a foam, usually in an aerosol, which makes it easy to distribute, and can be used on wet or dry hair. Mousses contain conditioning agents and proteins to nurture and protect the hair. They are available in different strengths, designed to give soft to maximum holding power, and can be used to lift flat roots or smooth frizz. Use when blow-drying, scrunching and diffuser-drying.
- **Volumizers and thickeners** help plump up flat or lifeless hair. Apply to damp hair before styling and focus on the roots rather than the lengths of the hair. They are often designed for fine hair, so are sold as a light formulation, perhaps as a lotion or light gel.
- **Gels** are styling aids that come in varying degrees of viscosity, from a thick jelly to a liquid spray, but will be heavier

Right *Different styling products do different things and you may find a blend of several offer the perfect solution for your needs.*

than a mousse or a blow-dry lotion. Gels are sometimes called sculpting lotions and are used for precise styling. They can be applied throughout the hair or to specific areas. Use them to lift roots, tame wisps and flyaways, create tendrils, calm static, heat set, and give structure and definition to curls. Wet gel can be used for sculpting styles which then dry to look slick.

- **Curl-activators or hair balms** are used to relax or straighten wavy or curly hair. They will often be delivered in pump-action sprays as light gels, which can then be easily distributed evenly by combing through the hair using a wide-toothed comb. The curl-activators (sometimes called a revitalizer) perk up curls by adding moisture to existing curls, helping renew their bounce.

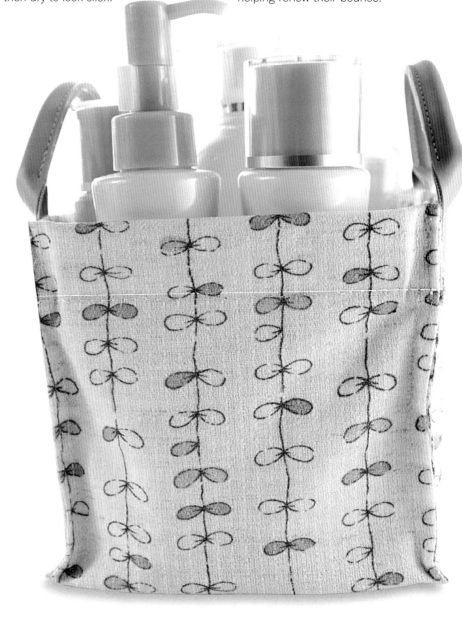

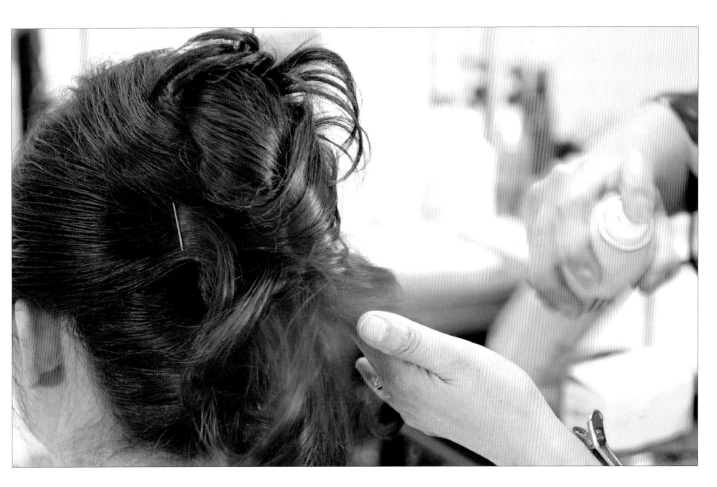

- **Heat-protective sprays and conditioning sprays and creams**
should be applied evenly throughout dry hair before using any heated styling tools including heated rollers, straightening irons, curling tongs or crimping irons. They form a barrier to protect the hair from excessive heat and so help prevent it being scorched or damaged.

Finish it
- **Hairspray** is traditionally used to hold a style in place and is available in varying degrees of stiffness to suit all needs. More creative uses include using hairspray to keep the hair in place, get curl definition when scrunching, and to mist over rollers when setting. Flexible or working sprays are also available and allow you to continue moving and shaping the hair after applying.

- **Serums, glossers, polishes and shine sprays** are made from oils or silicones, which improve shine and softness by forming a microscopic film on the surface of the hair. Formulations can vary from light and silky to heavier ones with a distinctly oily feel. They also contain substances designed to smooth the cuticle, encouraging the tiny scales to lie flat and thus reflect the light, and make the hair appear shiny.

Use these products to improve the feel of the hair, to combat static, de-frizz, add shine and gloss, and improve the appearance of split ends. Serum can be mixed with other products for extra-glossy drying or protection.

- **Waxes, pomades and creams** are made from natural waxes, such as carnauba (produced by

Left Products will be delivered as mousses, sprays, serums, gels and crèmes, depending on how they are to be applied.

Above Hairsprays are perfect for fixing an up-do once it is finished, while flexible or working sprays are used during styling.

a Brazilian palm tree), which are softened with other ingredients such as mineral oils and lanolin to make them pliable. They are designed to add definition and hold and both soft and hard formulations are available. Some pomades contain vegetable wax and oil to give gloss and sheen to hair. Other formulations produce foam and are water-soluble, and leave no residue. Use for dressing the hair, creating up-dos and for controlling frizz and static.

Did you know?

- *A light application of hairspray on a hairbrush can be used to tame flyaway ends.*
- *Use hairspray at the roots and tong or blow-dry the area to get immediate lift.*
- *A gel can be revitalized the following day by running wet fingers through the hair, against the direction of the finished look.*
- *If using a styling lotion for heat setting, look out for ones that offer thermal protection.*

Basic styling techniques

There are more ways to style hair than can possibly be outlined in one list, but here is a compilation of the most common techniques that form the basis for many more complex ways of dressing hair. It's all about practice making perfect!

Drying techniques

- **Finger-drying** hair creates gentle informal styles and is a technique that works well when your hair is well-behaved and inclined to fall into a style easily! It's great for drying shorter hair in particular, especially when you're not after a super-smooth finish.

Rather than using combs or brushes, your hands are the styling tools, lifting the hair and moving it in the direction you require, either allowing the hair to dry naturally or using a hairdryer on a low-power setting. You can mould the hair by wrapping it round your fingers, and push it to one side or back off your face.

- **Scrunch drying** is best for achieving fuller, more curly or textured styles on hair that already has some movement – usually medium or longer length. Take damp hair in the palm of your hand and compress it into a curled shape while directing the hairdryer on to the hair and opening and closing your hand to allow the heat into the hair. Keep your hand there until the hair cools and takes on the texture you want.

When the hair is dry and you want to finish the style, continue to scrunch the hair between the fingers and palm, adding styling mousse, gel or wax to help hold the shape.

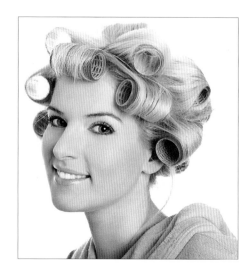

Above Using rollers is still arguably the best way to inject lift, volume and curl into hair of all types and lengths.

- **Natural drying** is a way of giving hair some respite from constant heat-styling. Hair is more elastic when it is wet, and when it is dried using a hairdryer and a brush or comb, the hair is stretched. Elastic recoil is delayed until the next time the hair is wet (either when it is shampooed or moisture is absorbed from the atmosphere). When dried naturally, however, the hair is not put under the duress of stretching, so has time to relax and regenerate.

Setting techniques

This refers to styling hair and putting it into a shape or texture that it doesn't naturally take on. It's a temporary process made possible by the fact that hair will take on moisture, allow itself to be reshaped and then dried or set into this new shape until next time it is dampened.

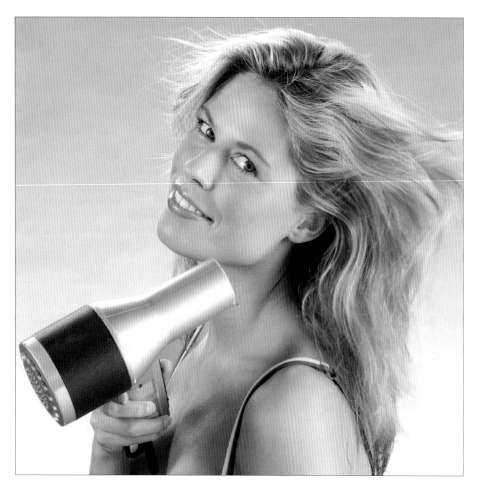

Left Heated styling tools need to be used with care as hair is easily scorched and scalps can be burned.

Setting techniques include curling, straightening, crimping and waving. These are all easily removed by simply washing the hair, returning it to its natural state.

Chemical processing

Sometimes called 'technical services', chemical processing uses chemicals to alter the state of the hair in a permanent or semi-permanent way. Broadly this refers to adding or removing colour, perming for curl, wave or volume, and relaxing to permanently straighten it.

Dressing hair

The art of folding, tying, wrapping and pinning hair into different shapes and designs, without cutting, setting or chemical processing is called dressing. Many styles comprise a technique or a combination of techniques based on the following:

- **Vertical rolls** (also called a pleat, French pleat or thumb roll) are created when hair is drawn off the head and held at a 90 degree angle, then wrapped around itself to form a barrel shape. You can use the fingers or whole hand to create the shape, depending on the size of roll you desire, and this is then pinned vertically against the head. You can form one large roll or use the technique to create smaller rolls.
- **Horizontal rolls** are formed the same way, but are pinned horizontally. They are a great way to accentuate the head shape, especially at the nape, the crown and the forehead.
- **Plaits**, also called braids, are strands of hair woven together. Usually, plaits are three strands of even sizes interwoven, but you can have five strands, and experiment with uneven-width strands.
- **Added hair** refers to wigs and hairpieces, which come in various shapes and sizes and can be made of synthetic fibre, monofibre or real hair. They come on different bases and can be clipped or pinned into your natural hair.
- **Extensions** are made from real or synthetic hair and are fixed or bonded into the root of your natural hair as close to the scalp as possible. They instantly extend the length and are useful for adding volume to fine or thinning hair. They are time-consuming to apply, but will last up to three months.

Common terms

When styling hair, certain parts of the head and neck will be referred to. Here's a guide to exactly where each part is:
- **The nape** is the lowest point of the head, where it joins the central point of the neck.
- **The crown** is the highest point of the head – towards the top back of the skull.
- **The forehead** is the point where hair is furthest forward.
- **The hairline** refers to the line where hair grows on the head.
- **The occipital bone** is the point on the back of the skull that sticks out furthest.

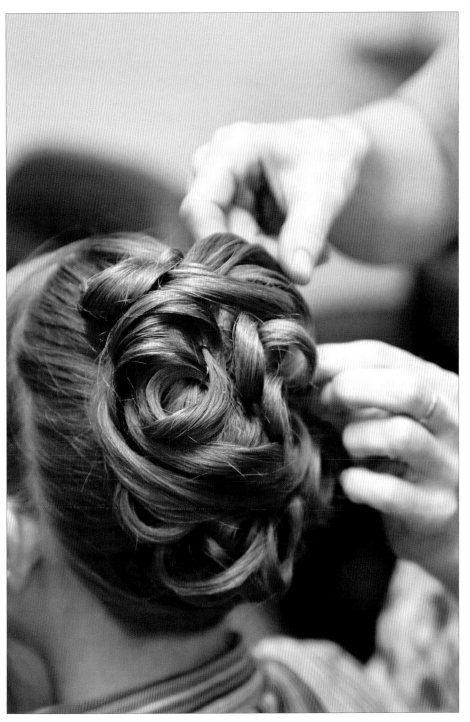

Left *It's tricky to see what's going on at the back when creating styles such as this, so get help with intricate styling and hairdressing.*

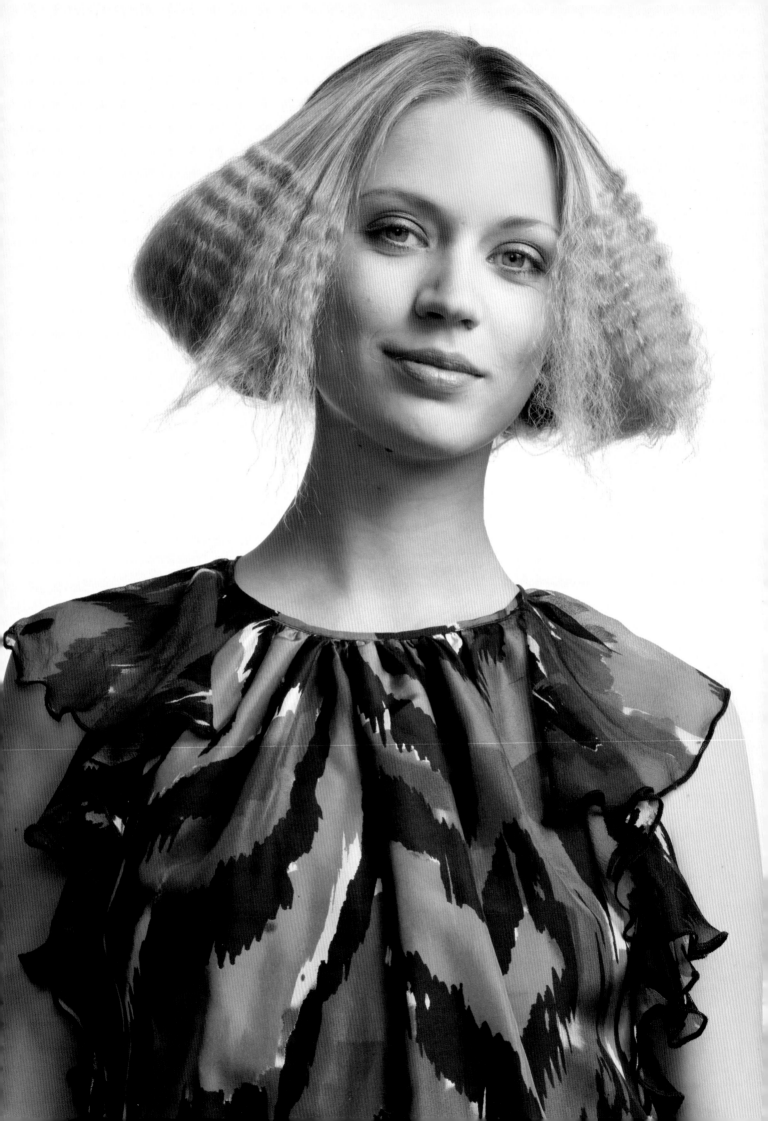

Everyday styling techniques

Once you have the right equipment for your hair, you need to master the art of styling it. This chapter is an invaluable step-by-step guide to some of the techniques that will enable you to create an almost endless number of looks – from blow-drying for different finishes to the correct way to use irons and tongs to create curls and waves. There are also step-by-step sequences for dressing your hair in a range of fantastic everyday styles, from soft finishes, ways to add texture and contrast and fringe (bangs) effects to up-dos, back-dos and pin-ups.

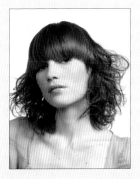 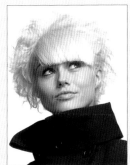 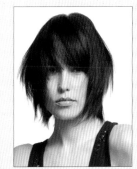

Blow-drying shorter hair for a smooth finish

For a really head-turning look that is easy to do, especially on one-length hair (whether short or long), go for a super-sleek finish. It creates shine to bring out the colour of the hair and complements a great head shape.

You will need
- Wide-tooth comb
- Lightweight holding gel
- Hairdryer
- Nozzle attachment
- Comb
- Paddle brush
- Shine spray

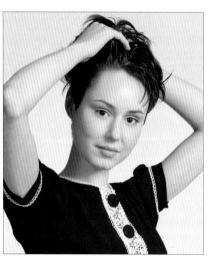

Stylist's note

Light bounces off smooth hair better than textured hair, which is why this finish achieves greater shine.

1 Wash your hair, then towel-dry it to be damp rather than wet. Comb through to detangle using a wide-tooth comb, which won't stretch and break your hair.

2 Apply a lightweight gel and work through your hair using your fingers so it is evenly distributed from roots to ends.

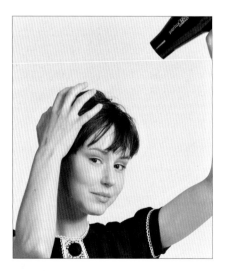

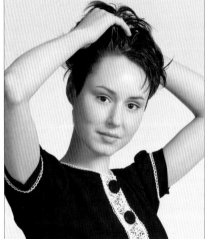

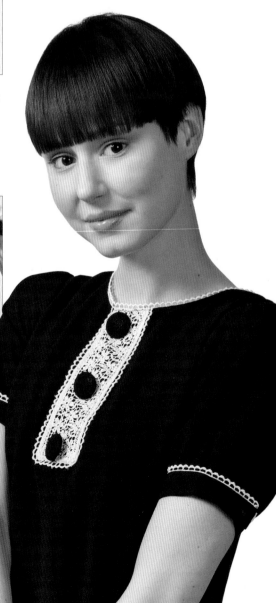

3 Rough-dry your hair with a hairdryer to be about 80 per cent dry, then style as you like using a comb.

4 Brush your hair from root to end with a paddle brush, following with the hairdryer. Spritz all over with shine spray to finish.

Blow-drying shorter hair smooth with kicked-out ends

Using a brush when blow-drying gives you a super-smooth finish, but remember you can also use it to kick out the ends of the hair. It makes for a refreshing change from straight or curled-under bobbed looks.

You will need

- Wide-tooth comb
- Texturizing product
- Hairdryer
- Nozzle attachment
- Large round brush

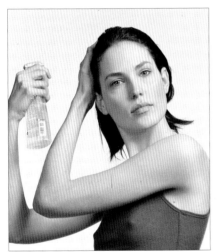

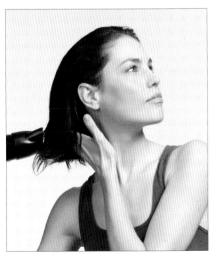

Stylist's note

For speed, blow-dry your hair roughly until it is 80 per cent dry before taking more time to smooth the hair by styling with a hairbrush as you finish drying it.

1 Wash your hair, then towel-dry it to be damp. Comb through to detangle using a wide-tooth comb. Apply a texturizer, such as a light-hold gel product.

2 Work the gel through your hair from roots to ends, using your fingers to ensure it is evenly distributed.

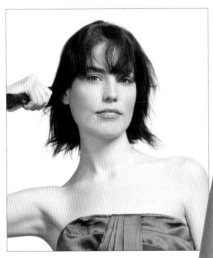

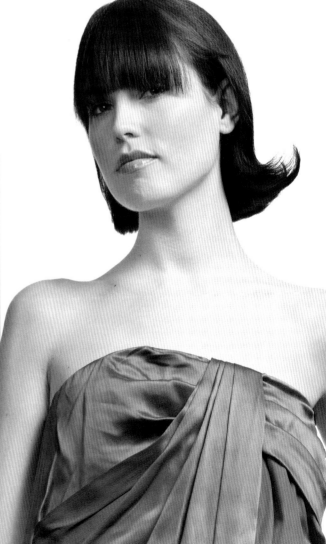

3 Rough-dry your hair with a hairdryer, using your fingers to help lift at the roots.

4 Use a large round brush to wrap sections of hair round the bristles, then roll the brush outwards and blast-dry to create a kick at the ends of your hair.

Blow-drying shorter hair for a chic, grown-up look

Short hair doesn't have to be worn close and flat to your head. By using a variety of hairbrushes to lift the hair at the roots as you blow-dry, it's easy to create a smooth yet full-looking style that is neat and chic at the same time.

Stylist's note

Using a small-barrelled round brush won't necessarily create curl; it can also be used for adding root lift and volume.

1 Wash your hair, then towel-dry it to be damp rather than wet. Comb through to detangle using a wide-tooth comb, which won't stretch and break your hair.

2 Spritz your hair all over with styling spray to prevent scorching hair when drying it.

3 Blow-dry your hair by wrapping sections round a small-barrelled round brush then lifting and rolling it inwards to achieve smoothness and volume as you dry.

4 Smooth your hair back off your face using a vent brush to create a wedge at the nape of your neck. Spritz with hairspray to finish.

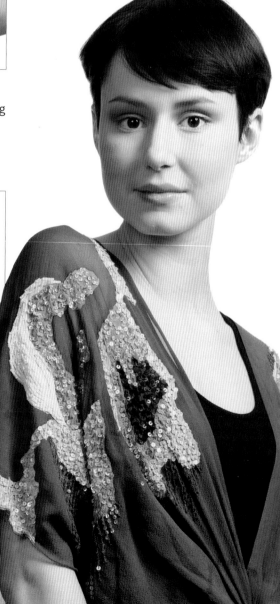

Blow-drying shorter hair for a sleek, shiny finish

Even with dynamic, choppy layers cut into shorter hair, you can still choose to wear a smooth style to accentuate great condition, colour and shape. Use a flat brush to keep hair close to the head and looking sleek.

You will need
- Wide-tooth comb
- Styling lotion
- Hairdryer
- Nozzle attachment
- Flat brush
- Hairspray

Stylist's note

Once styled, you can spritz hairspray on to the hairbrush and run it through your hair to calm flyaways.

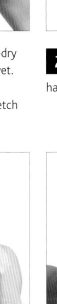

1 Wash your hair, then towel-dry it to be damp rather than wet. Comb through to detangle using a wide-tooth comb, which won't stretch and break your hair.

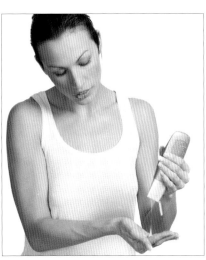

2 Tip some styling lotion into the palm of one hand, then rub your hands together.

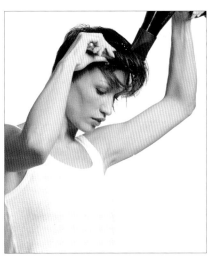

3 Rub the styling lotion through the hair using your hands. Ensure it is evenly distributed from root to tip.

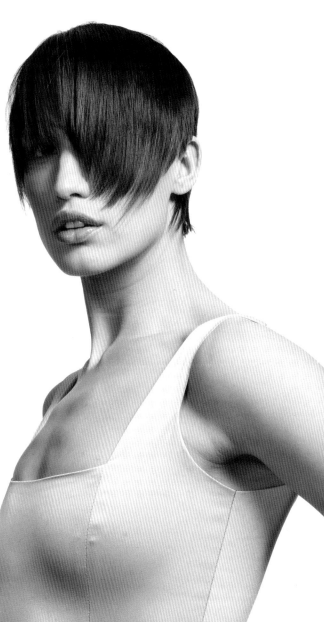

4 Blow-dry your hair smooth using a flat brush to keep layers close to the head. Style to show off the cut. Spritz with hairspray to finish.

Blow-drying the perfect long bob

A sleek, swinging bob is a timeless look that never goes out of fashion. Whether yours is cut with or without a fringe, and whatever the length of hair, blow-dry a bob smooth for maximum shine and impact.

You will need
- Wide-tooth comb
- Sectioning clips
- Large round brush
- Hairdryer
- Nozzle attachment
- Shine spray

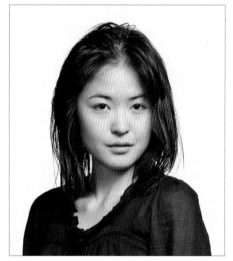

1 Wash your hair, then towel-dry it to be damp rather than wet. Comb through to detangle using a wide-tooth comb, which won't stretch and break your hair.

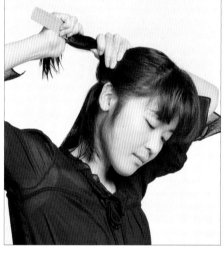

2 Section hair from mid-forehead to centre back and across the occipital bone from ear to ear.

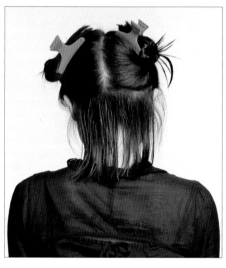

3 The back sectioning should now look like this.

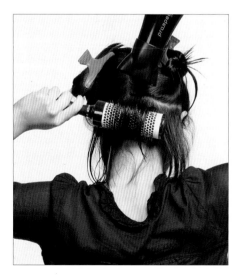

4 Starting at the back, place a large, round brush near the roots and hold a dryer with nozzle attachment above the hair.

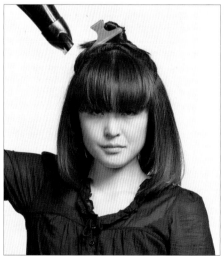

5 Work round the lower section of your hair before moving to the upper section.

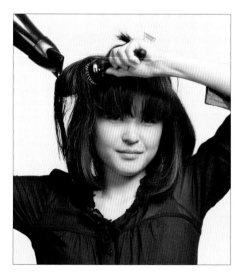

6 Now dry the upper section, continuing to wrap hair round the large round brush for a smooth finish.

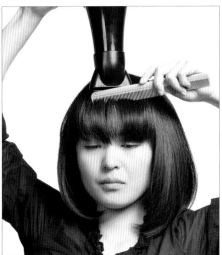

7 Blow-dry the fringe (bangs) area using a comb rather than a hairbrush for a smooth but flatter finish.

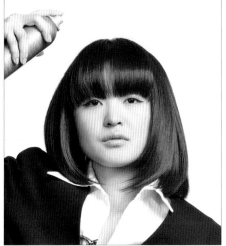

8 Spritz hair with a light-hold shine spray for a great look.

Stylist's note

This style requires healthy-looking hair, so maintain great condition, and be wary of over-drying, which can cause hair to frizz.

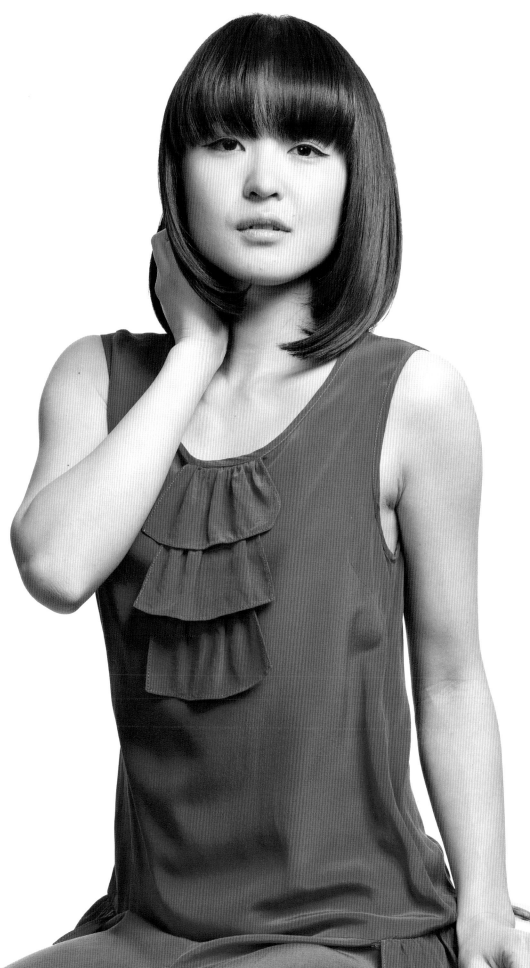

Blow-drying shorter hair for a soft, relaxed look

Giving a shorter haircut a gently dishevelled finish softens a look without making it too sweet or cute. This is an easy-to-achieve and relaxed look that will flatter a strong jawline or a square face shape.

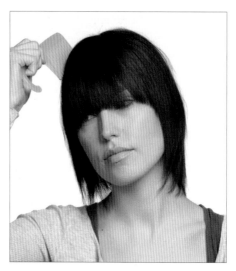

1 Wash your hair, then towel or blow-dry it so it is completely dry.

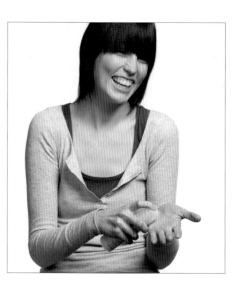

2 Comb through hair with a wide-tooth comb to eliminate tangles.

3 Put some moulding paste in your palm and rub your hands together, allowing the paste to warm through. This makes it easier to apply.

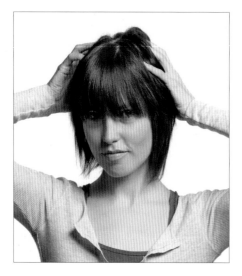

4 Using your fingers, work the paste through your hair from roots to ends for even coverage and maximum texture and volume.

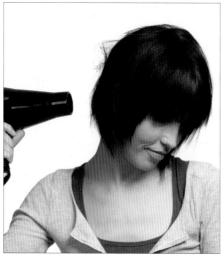

5 Blast your hair with a hairdryer, focusing particularly on roots for lift and movement.

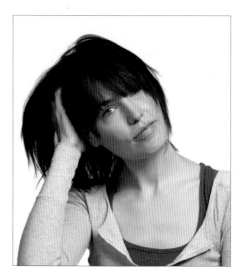

6 Shake your head and run your fingers through your hair to loosen up the hair.

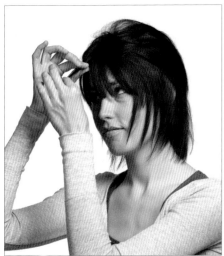

7 Put some defining wax on your fingertips and rub through pieces of hair to enhance texture.

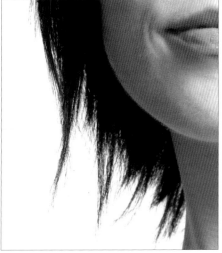

8 The perimeter of the hair should look shattered, like this. Spritz your hair with shine spray to finish.

Stylist's note

Stiffer products such as moulding pastes are best warmed in the hands to make them more pliable and easier to apply evenly.

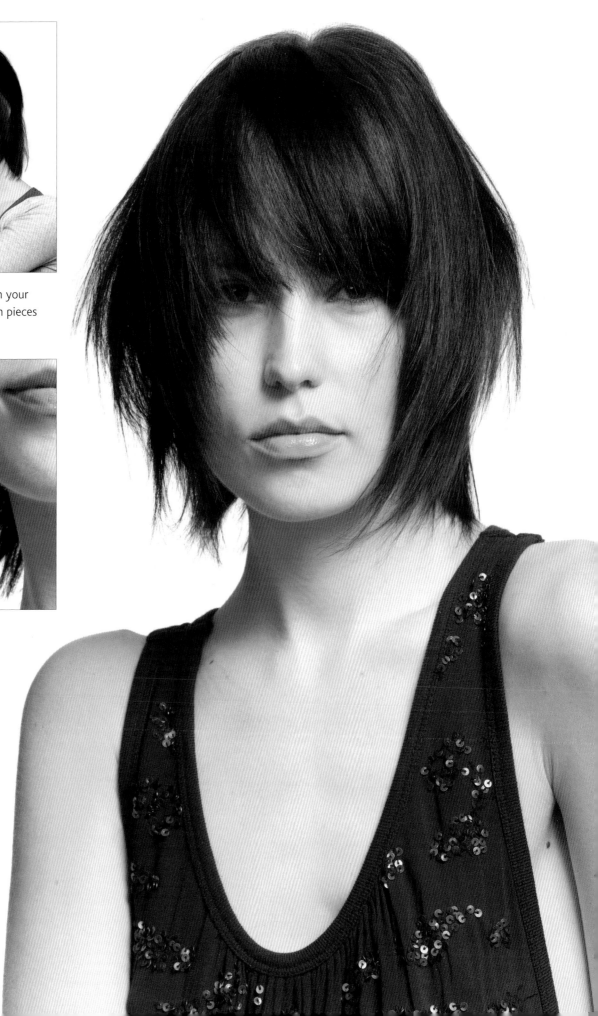

Blow-drying shorter hair for a multi-texture effect

You will need
- Hairbrush
- Comb
- Heat-protective spray
- Straightening irons
- Hairspray

Using a combination of straightening irons and styling products you can create a fabulous style that is wearable and striking at the same time. It's fun to play with different textures and contrasts, so let your imagination run wild.

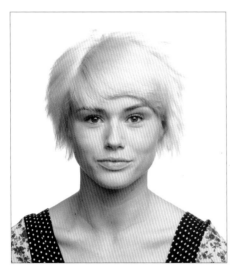

1 Brush clean, dry hair to be tangle-free, then put it in a diagonal front parting, as shown.

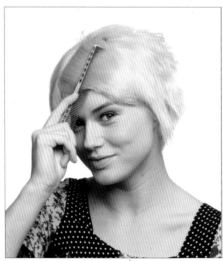

2 Comb through the front section so it is really smooth.

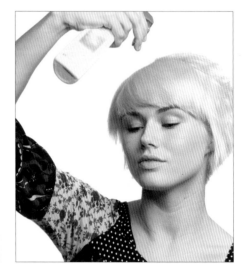

3 Spritz your hair all over with heat-protective spray to prevent scorching hair when straightening it.

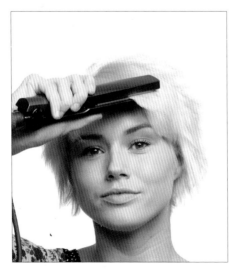

4 Apply straightening irons through the front section, working from the roots to the ends, to make it as smooth as possible.

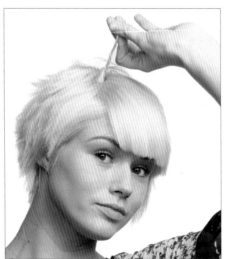

5 Taking one small section at a time from the rest of your hair, twist the hair upwards with your fingers.

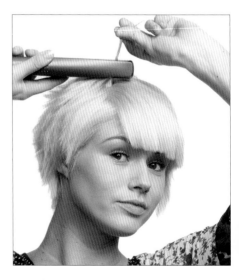

6 Clamp the twist between the plates of the straightening irons, hold for 5 seconds and release.

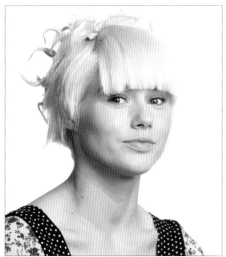

7 Continue to work small sections over the whole head in the same way, but always leaving out the smooth front section.

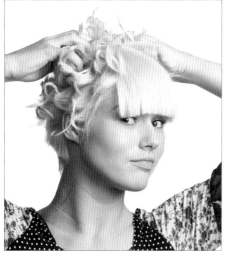

8 Using the fingers, loosen the twists slightly so they blend together, then spritz all over with hairspray for hold.

Stylist's note

Clamping twists of hair in the straightening irons ensures that the texture will remain fixed until you wash it out.

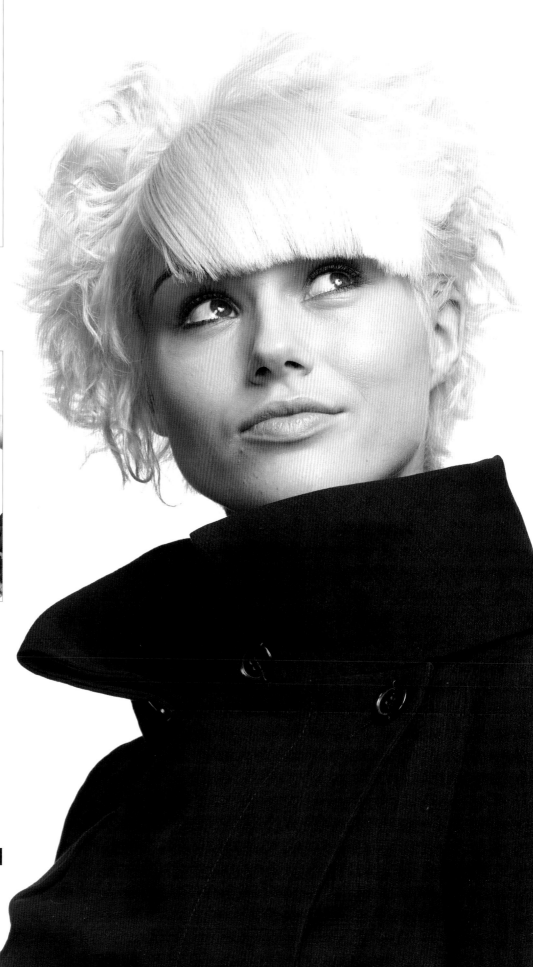

Blow-drying shorter hair for a textured finish

When time is of the essence, working with the natural texture and movement of shorter hair is a fast way to achieve a great look that will appear to have taken longer to create than it really has. Fantastic!

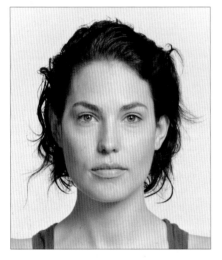

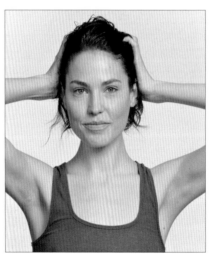

Stylist's note

Invest in an ionic hairdryer, which won't suck all the moisture out of the hair, leaving it in better condition and reducing static and frizz.

1 Wash your hair, then towel-dry it to be damp rather than wet. Comb through to detangle using a wide-tooth comb, which won't stretch and break your hair.

2 Apply a texturizing product to your hair and evenly distribute it through using your fingers. The thicker the product, the more textured the hair will appear.

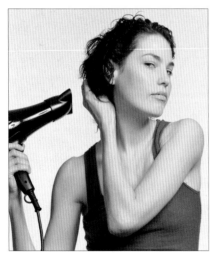

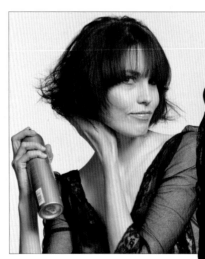

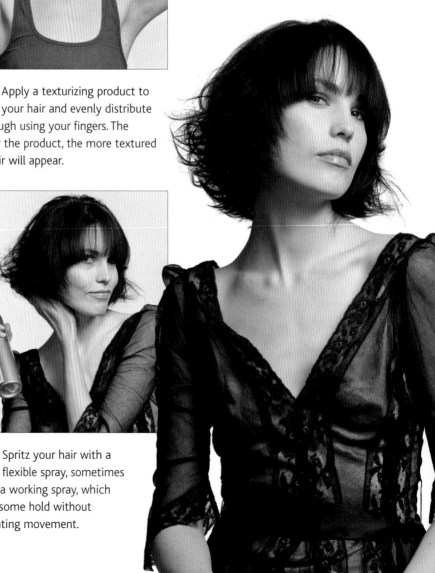

3 Holding the hairdryer at least 6cm/2½in away from your hair (to avoid scorching), blast-dry, using your fingers to keep shaping the hair and to prevent tangles forming.

4 Spritz your hair with a flexible spray, sometimes called a working spray, which offers some hold without preventing movement.

Blow-drying to add contrast to a shorter textured style

Working smooth sections into a textured hairstyle can be very striking and create an individual finish that is fun yet smart or chic at the same time. Use a shine spray to emphasize the contrast between the smooth and more choppy textures.

You will need

- Comb
- Styling mousse
- Hairdryer
- Nozzle attachment
- Flat brush
- Smoothing crème
- Hairspray

Stylist's note

For a smoother back area and more choppy front, simply reverse the process, always using the fingers to create texture where you want it, but working hair around a brush for sleeker finishes.

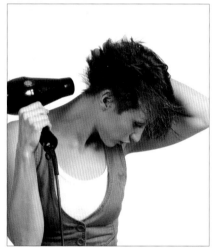

1 Wash your hair, then towel-dry it to be damp rather than wet. Comb through to detangle. Apply styling mousse throughout, using your fingers and ensuring it is evenly distributed.

2 Rough-dry the main part of your hair with a hairdryer, using your fingers to achieve maximum texture and movement.

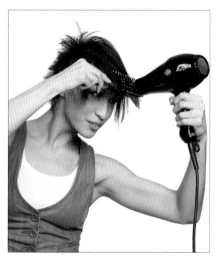

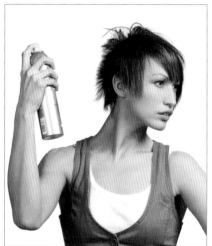

3 Smooth out the front section by blow-drying it, using a flat brush to emphasize different layers in the hair.

4 Sweep the front section to one side, slick on a small amount of smoothing crème and spritz with light-hold spray to fix hair in position.

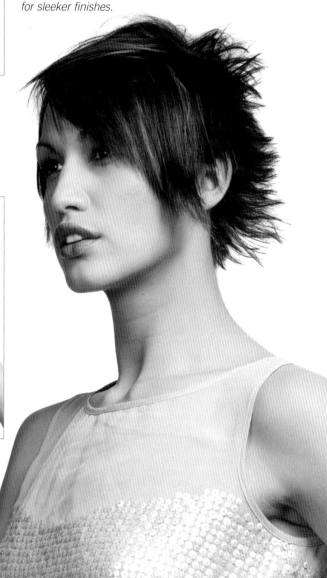

Blow-drying to add volume and choppy texture to shorter hair

A choppy finish to a short haircut instantly adds individuality to your look. Make the style as exuberant as you like and emphasize layers and colours in the hair by applying a wax or defining spray and shaping with your fingers.

You will need
- Wide-tooth comb
- Light-hold gel
- Hairdryer
- Nozzle attachment
- Medium-hold hairspray
- Defining wax

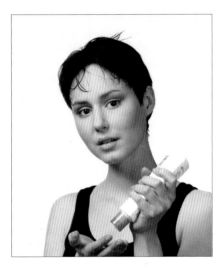

1 Wash your hair, then towel-dry it to be damp. Detangle using a wide-tooth comb, which won't stretch and break your hair. Squeeze some light-hold gel into the palm of your hand.

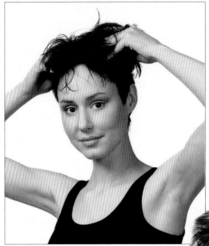

2 Massage the gel into your hair using your fingers, ensuring it is distributed evenly from root to tip.

Stylist's note

A heavily textured finish is a fantastic way to bring out the different highlights in your hair.

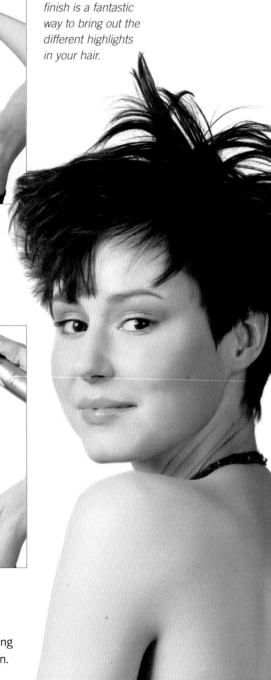

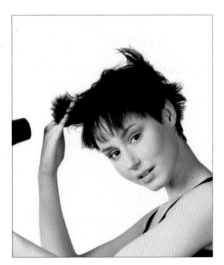

3 Rough-dry your hair using a hairdryer, lifting the hair to direct heat specifically at the roots.

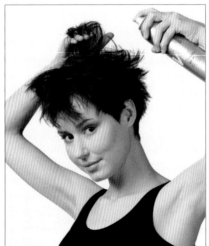

4 Spray the roots with a medium-hold hairspray for height, volume and staying power. Apply a defining wax to finish, piecing it through the ends to add definition.

Blow-drying mid-length hair for all-over texture

Creating texture all over your hair doesn't mean going wild. Use a small-barrelled round brush to imbue your hair with movement and softness that is smart-looking yet relaxed too, and which won't look as though you've tried so hard.

You will need
- Wide-tooth comb
- Texturizing spray
- Hairdryer
- Nozzle attachment
- Small-barrelled round brush
- Hairspray

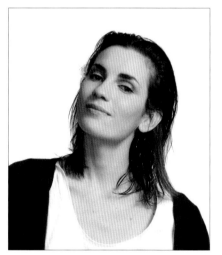

Stylist's note

Break up a blocky fringe (bangs) by sweeping it to one side, or pushing it up, and blast-drying the roots with a hairdryer for height and hold.

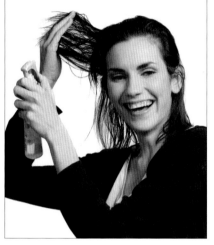

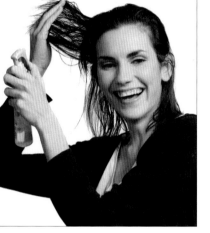

1 Wash your hair, then towel-dry it to be damp rather than wet. Comb through to detangle using a wide-tooth comb, which won't stretch and break your hair.

2 Spritz your hair with texturizing spray directed at the roots for lift and then at the mid-lengths to add volume.

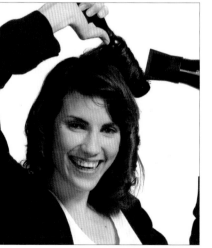

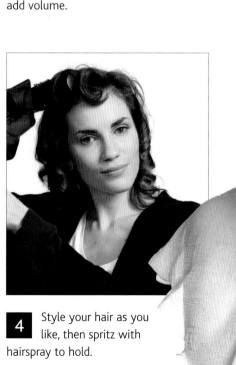

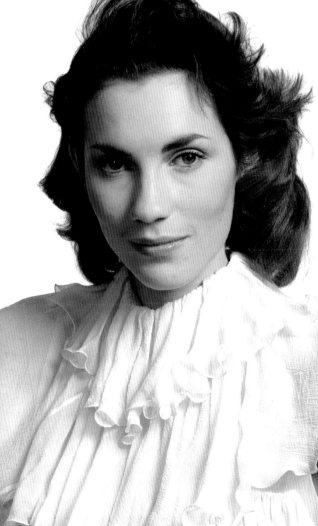

3 Rough-dry the hair with a hairdryer, then work round the head wrapping irregular sections of hair round a small-barrelled round brush and drying into shape.

4 Style your hair as you like, then spritz with hairspray to hold.

Blow-drying fringed mid-length hair for a textured finish

Have a little fun and create a vibrant, natural look with movement and style that brings out your individuality. Contrasting a smooth fringe with the rest of the hair prevents this look from becoming too casual.

You will need
- Wide-tooth comb
- Texturizing styling spray
- Hairdryer
- Nozzle attachment
- Hairbrush

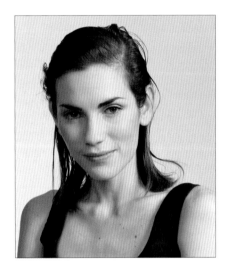

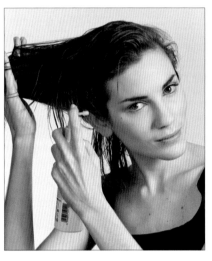

Stylist's note

There are plenty of great texturizing products that you can experiment with. A spray is easy to apply, especially when you are focusing on one area in particular.

1 Wash your hair, then towel-dry it to be damp rather than wet. Comb through to detangle using a wide-tooth comb, which won't stretch and break your hair.

2 Spritz a texturizing spray on the roots of your hair to help create lift when drying.

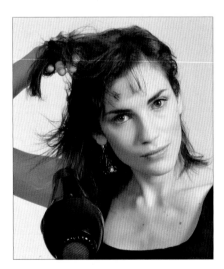

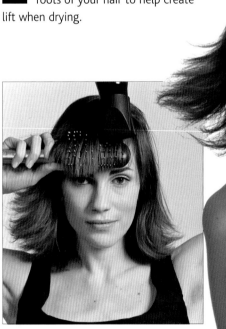

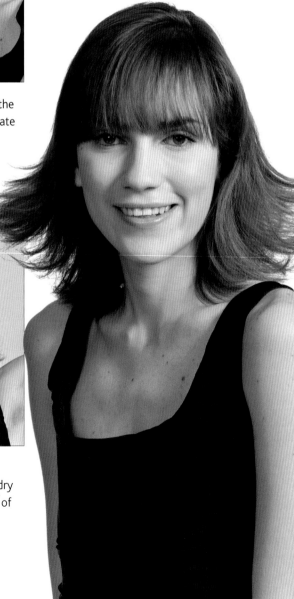

3 Blast-dry your hair with a hairdryer, directing heat at the roots to create volume and using your fingers to lift your hair for a less polished finish.

4 Wrap the fringe (bangs) area round a hairbrush and blow-dry it smooth for contrast with the rest of your hair.

Blow-drying mid-length or longer hair for a loose finish

Use this simple technique to achieve a clean, natural finish that doesn't look forced or overdone. Quick and easy to do, it will enable you to be ready and heading for the door super-quickly, safe in the knowledge that your hair looks amazing.

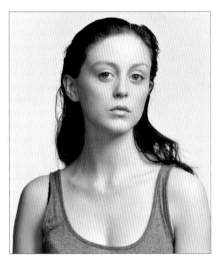

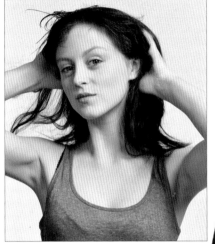

Stylist's note

Point the hairdryer so the warm air only flows down the length of the hair, helping smooth the cuticles to create shine.

1 Wash your hair, then towel-dry it to be damp rather than wet. Comb through to detangle using a wide-tooth comb, which won't stretch and break your hair.

2 Apply a smoothing product such as a light balm to your hair using your fingers, paying particular attention to the mid-lengths and ends rather than the roots.

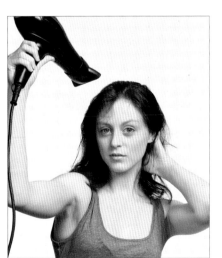

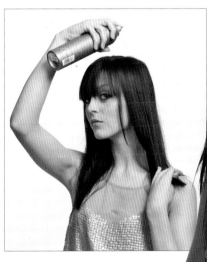

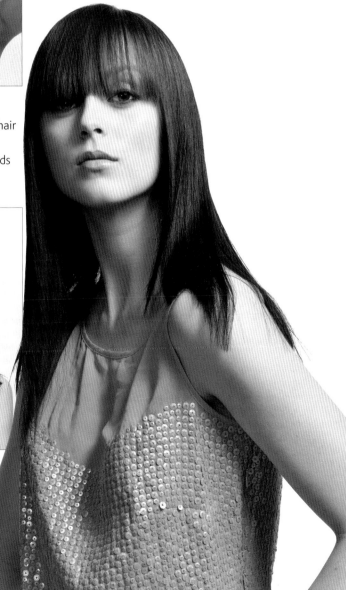

3 Holding the dryer at least 6cm/2½in away from your hair (to avoid scorching), dry the hair, running your fingers through the lengths to prevent tangles forming.

4 Apply a light-hold shine spray all over to finish.

Blow-drying mid-length or longer hair to curl under

A neat, classic finish that works best on longer or mid-length hair that has either no layers or just simple graduation, this is a perfect wear-anywhere style that will take you from home to the office and on to the dance-floor, looking good every time.

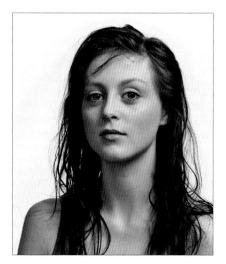

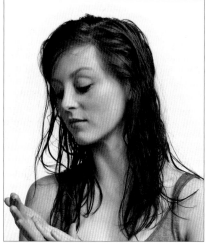

Stylist's note

Using a large round brush to finish the styling achieves a better curl than a flatter brush can.

1 Wash your hair, then towel-dry it to be damp rather than wet. Comb through to detangle using a wide-tooth comb, which won't stretch and break your hair.

2 Put some styling serum in the palm of one hand, then rub your hands together.

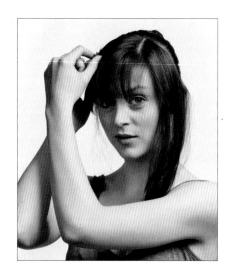

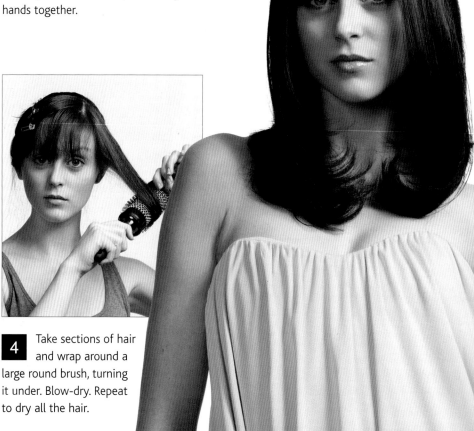

3 Rub the serum through your hair from root to tip, distributing the product evenly. Section off one side, twisting and clipping it out of the way with sectioning clips until needed.

4 Take sections of hair and wrap around a large round brush, turning it under. Blow-dry. Repeat to dry all the hair.

Blow-drying mid-length or longer hair for a bedhead finish

Shake up your style by moving away from the groomed look and instead adding as much texture as possible to your hair's natural movement. This works particularly well for shorter or mid-length cuts that have some layering.

You will need
- Wide-tooth comb
- Volumizing mousse
- Hairdryer
- Hairspray

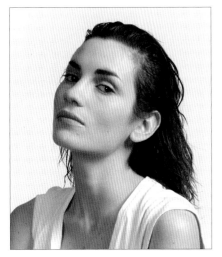

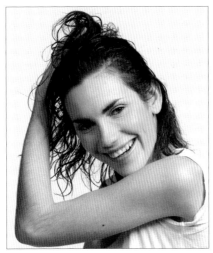

Stylist's note

Avoid creating 'holes' in the style by keeping the hairdryer moving and not lingering too long on one spot.

1 Wash your hair, then towel-dry it to be damp rather than wet. Comb through to detangle using a wide-tooth comb, which won't stretch and break your hair.

2 Squirt some volumizing mousse into the palm of your hand and apply it liberally throughout the hair for body and volume. Ensure it is evenly distributed from root to tip.

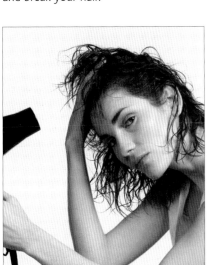

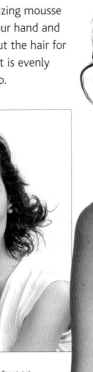

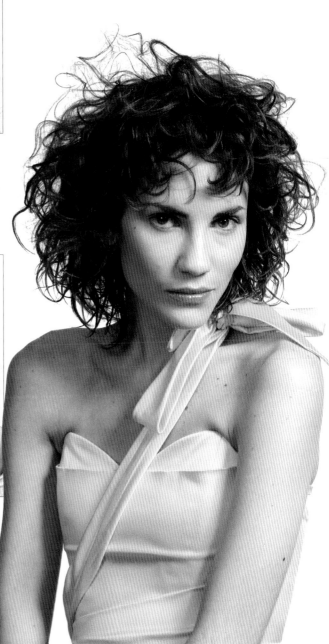

3 Blast-dry the hair by continually moving the hairdryer swiftly around the head but focusing particularly on the roots to add lift.

4 Scrunch the hair between your fingers and palm to add texture and lift as the hair dries. Spritz all over with hairspray to hold the style.

Blow-drying longer hair for a smooth finish

You will need
- Wide-tooth comb
- Styling mousse
- Sectioning clips
- Bristle brush
- Hairdryer
- Nozzle attachment
- Shine spray

Long hair looks sensational when it moves with a shiny, healthy swing, so take a little more time than usual when blow-drying to maximize a sleek finish. It's well worth the effort, and is easier than you think to achieve.

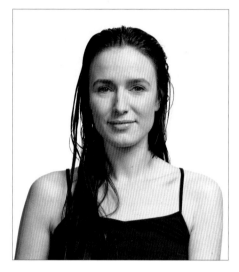

1 Wash your hair, then towel-dry it to be damp rather than wet. Comb through to detangle using a wide-tooth comb, which won't stretch and break your hair.

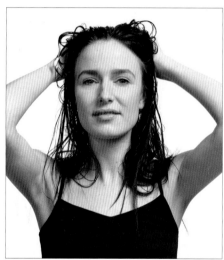

2 Squirt some mousse into the palm of your hand, then rub your hands together and apply the mousse to the mid-lengths and ends of your hair.

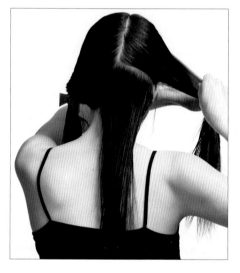

3 Section the hair, twisting and clipping the upper and side pieces out of the way with sectioning clips. Ensure the front parting is where you will want it to be when you finish blow-drying the hair.

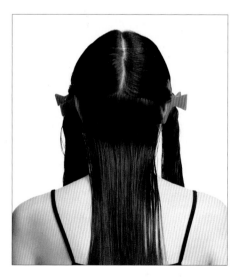

4 When the hair has been sectioned, the back of your head should look like this, with the hair at the back ready to be dried first.

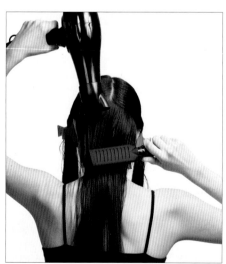

5 Starting at the back, place a bristle brush near the roots and hold a hairdryer so the nozzle points down along the length of the hair.

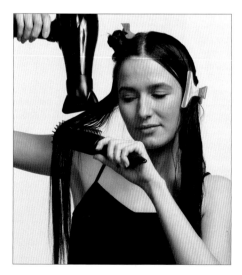

6 Keep drawing the brush through the section of hair, following with the hairdryer, holding it at least 6cm/2in from the hair to prevent scorching.

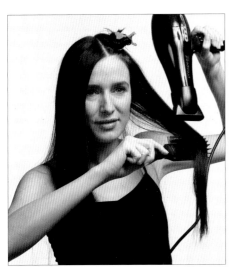

7 When the back is dry, work around the sides of the head, drying one section at a time in the same way.

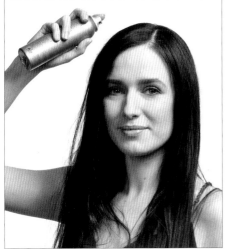

8 When all the hair is dry and smooth, spritz all over with a light shine spray to finish.

Stylist's note

Using sectioning clips makes it easier to work through the hair systematically and achieve a professional-looking finish.

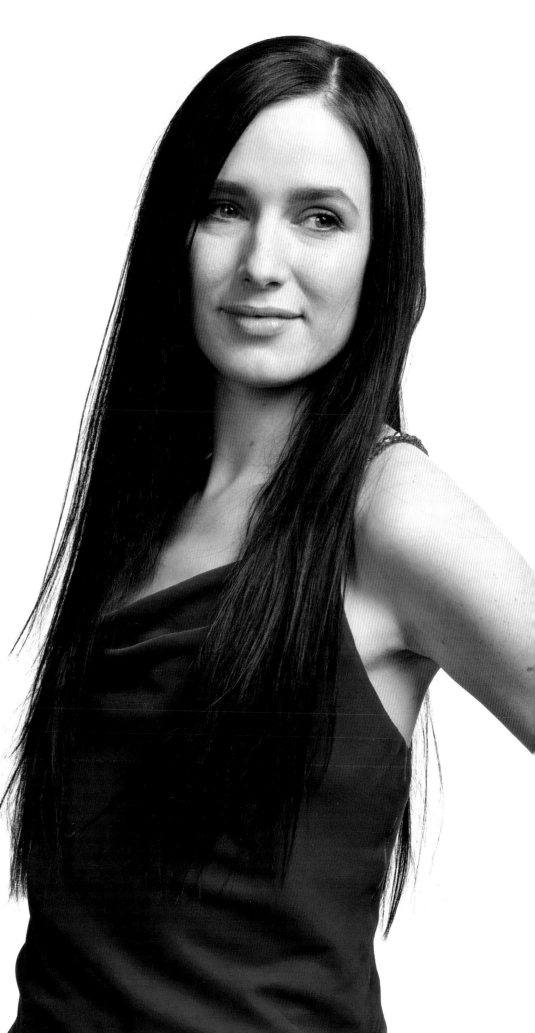

Blow-drying longer hair for volume and movement

Fixing a diffuser attachment onto the hairdryer is a great way to achieve volume and natural texture on longer hair. Easy to achieve, this technique is a gentle way to enhance fullness and movement for a luxurious, head-turning finish.

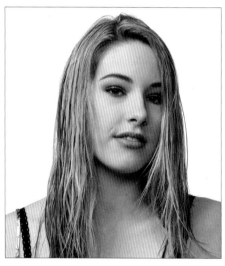

1 Wash your hair, then towel-dry it to be damp rather than wet. Comb through to detangle using a wide-tooth comb, which won't stretch and break your hair.

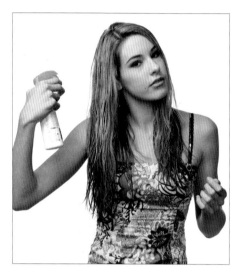

2 Spritz your hair all over with a heat-protective spray to prevent scorching hair when drying it.

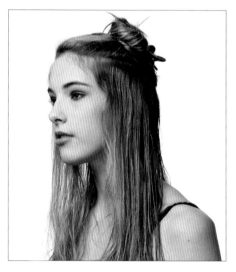

3 Section off the top area, twisting and clipping it out of the way with sectioning clips until needed.

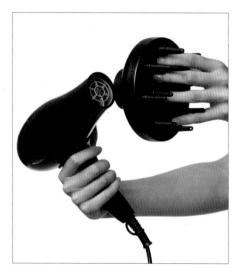

4 Fix the diffuser attachment to the end of the hairdryer.

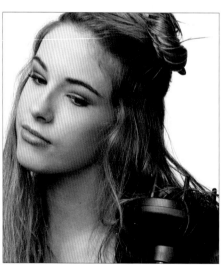

5 Position the diffuser under the ends and mid-lengths of your hair (it can touch the hair) and select a cool- to mid-heat temperature.

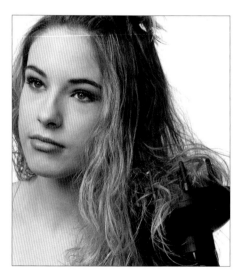

6 Work around your head drying your hair in sections, ensuring it rests on the diffuser, to help maximize texture.

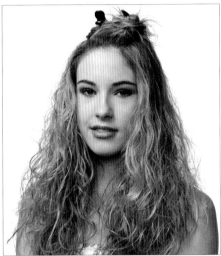

7 When you have finished the lower sections should have plenty of texture and volume.

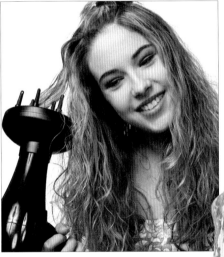

8 Remove the sectioning clips and work through the top section of hair in the same way, until all your hair is completely dry.

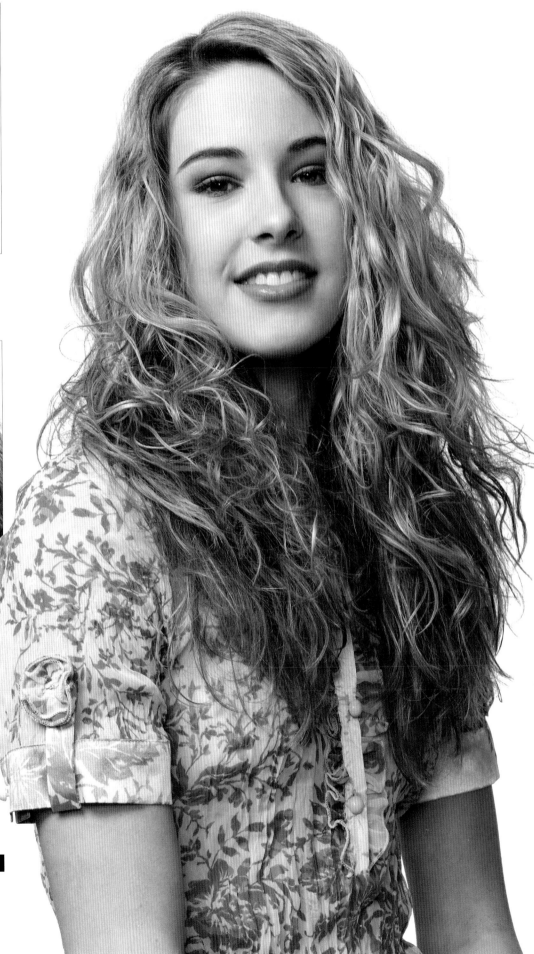

Blow-drying curly hair for a soft, smooth look

It's possible to achieve a smooth look even on naturally very curly hair. Use your expertise with blow-drying to straighten the hair, then tame movement using straightening irons and styling products for a fantastic finish.

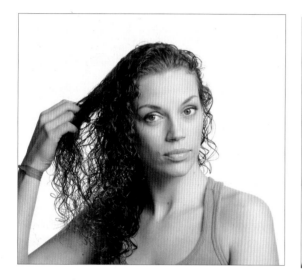

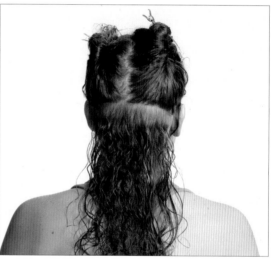

1 Wash your hair, then towel-dry it to be damp. Comb through to detangle using a wide-tooth comb, which won't stretch and break your hair. Apply styling lotion hair using your fingers to ensure it is distributed evenly from root to end.

2 Section your hair into three parts using sectioning clips, as shown. This will make drying and straightening your hair easier.

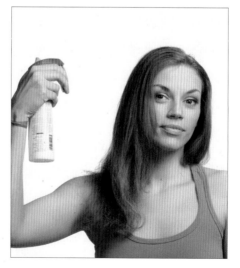

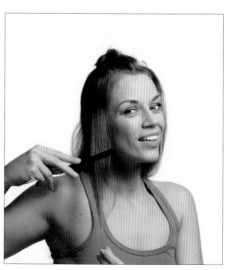

3 Working through the sections, blow-dry the hair by wrapping it round a large-barrelled brush to achieve as smooth a finish as possible

4 Spritz your hair all over with heat-protective spray.

5 Section your hair again into three parts. Comb your hair to ensure it is tangle-free.

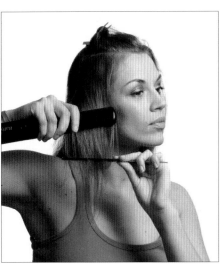

6 Apply straightening irons to each section in turn, working from root to end.

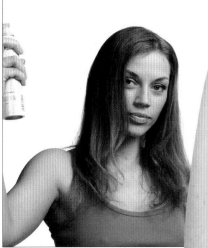

7 Apply shine spray and serum to your hair for a super-sleek finish.

Stylist's note

Don't cut corners by skipping the smooth blow-dry as part of this technique. Applying straightening irons to curly hair just won't deliver a sleek result.

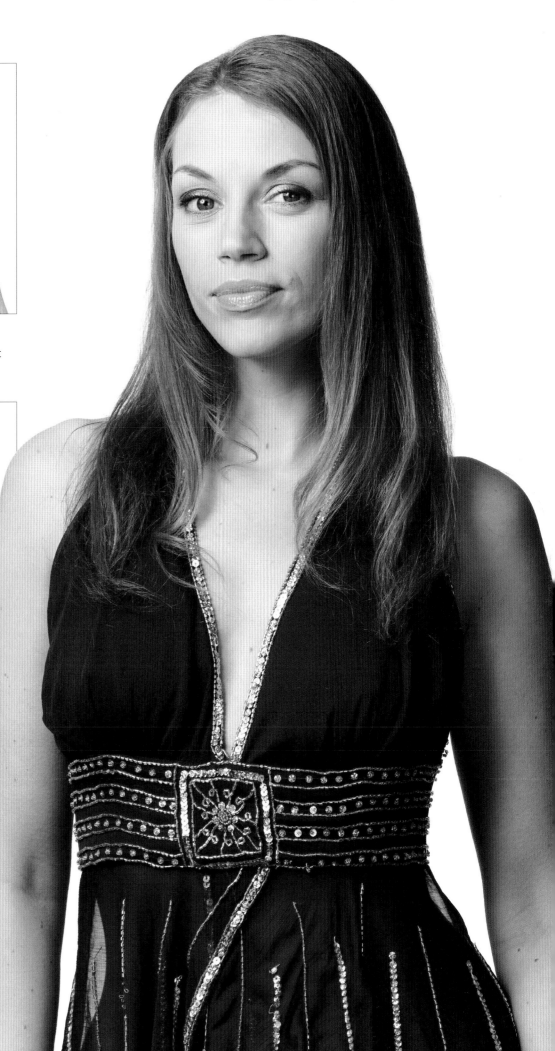

Blow-drying to add emphasis to a deep, wide fringe

Accentuating a strong or noticeable feature of a haircut, such as a deep fringe, creates a striking look. Contrast the texture of the fringe with the rest of your hair to create emphasis, using different styling products and tools.

You will need
- Wide-tooth comb
- Styling mousse
- Hairdryer
- Nozzle attachment
- Small-barrelled round brush
- Hairspray

Stylist's note

To apply hairspray, hold the can above your head so that the spray settles on to your hair as it falls.

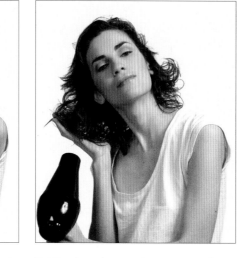

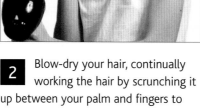

1 Wash your hair, then towel-dry it to be damp rather than wet. Comb through to detangle. Apply styling mousse throughout, using your fingers and ensuring it is evenly distributed.

2 Blow-dry your hair, continually working the hair by scrunching it up between your palm and fingers to create texture.

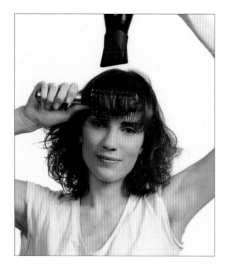

3 Dry the fringe (bangs) area smooth by wrapping the hair round a small-barrelled brush and brushing downwards, lifting the hair as you go, while drying.

4 Spritz hair with a light-hold spray to finish and smooth the front section using the palm of the hand to calm flyaways.

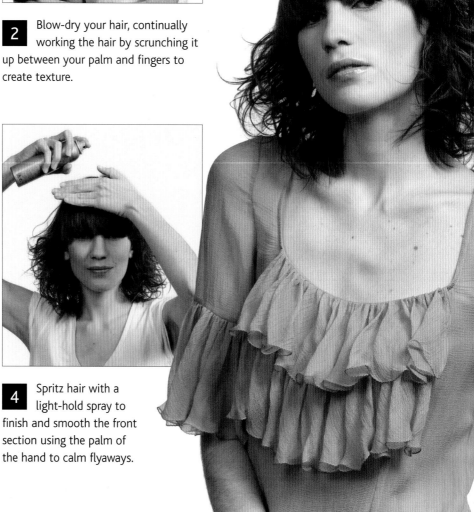

Tonging shorter hair for texture

You will need
- Heat-protective spray
- Small-barrelled tongs
- Styling wax

For a more groomed yet texturized finish that doesn't involve rough-drying or back-combing, practise using tongs. As long as there is enough length to wrap hair once around the barrel then you can achieve a great look this way.

Stylist's note

If sections of your hair are too short to wrap around the tongs, leave this hair free and work with longer sections only.

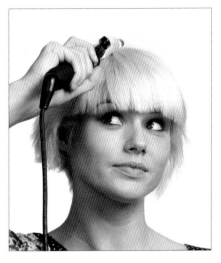

1 Spritz dry, clean hair all over with heat-protective spray to prevent scorching hair when tonging it.

2 Taking one small section of hair at a time, place the tongs at the end of the hair and wind up to the roots. Hold for a few seconds.

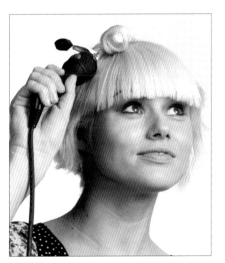

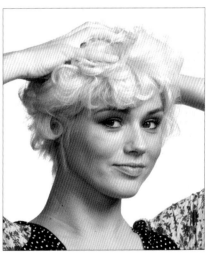

3 This technique forms small half-curls, as shown. Work around the entire head in the same way, including a fringe (bangs) area.

4 To finish, gently loosen the curls with your fingers (not a hairbrush) and apply a small amount of styling wax to separate and define the texture.

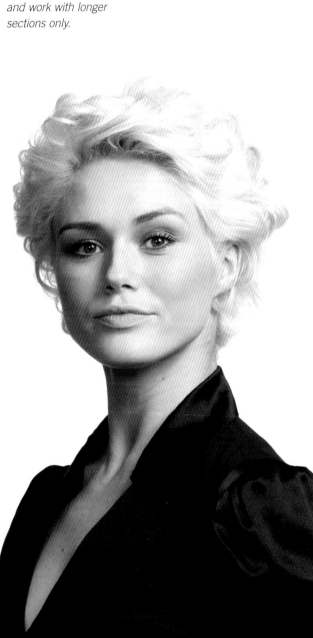

Using tongs for different curled effects

Practise using curling tongs in different ways to create all types of curl, including ringlets and spiral winds. Tongs are a fantastically versatile styling tool once you have the know-how and you can choose ones with different-size barrels to suit.

You will need
- Comb
- Heat-protective spray
- Curling tongs
- Hairspray

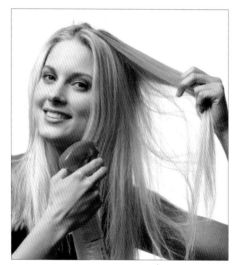

1 Comb through clean, dry hair so that it is tangle-free.

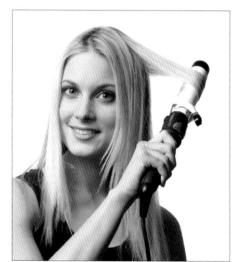

2 Spritz your hair all over with a heat-protective spray to prevent the tongs from scorching or drying out your hair.

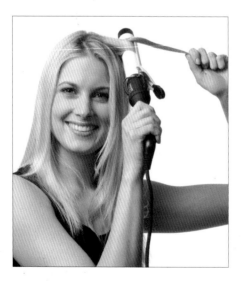

3 Working with a small section of hair at a time, place the tongs at the end and wind back up to the root. Hold for a few seconds, then release. Repeat the action with all of your hair.

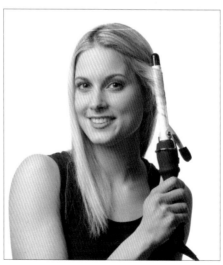

4 Alternatively, for a softer curl, place the tongs near the root and wrap the hair round the barrel of the tongs until you reach the end.

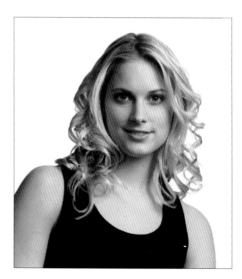

5 For a spiral wind, using small-barrelled tongs, take smaller sections of hair and wind from the ends up to the roots while holding the tongs vertically.

6 This is how a spiral wind finish looks when it has been applied to the whole head.

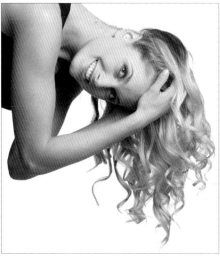

7 When all your hair is curled as you want it, tip your head upside down and shake to loosen curls.

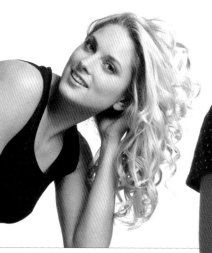

8 If desired, loosen again by running your fingers through the hair, then spritz with hairspray for hold.

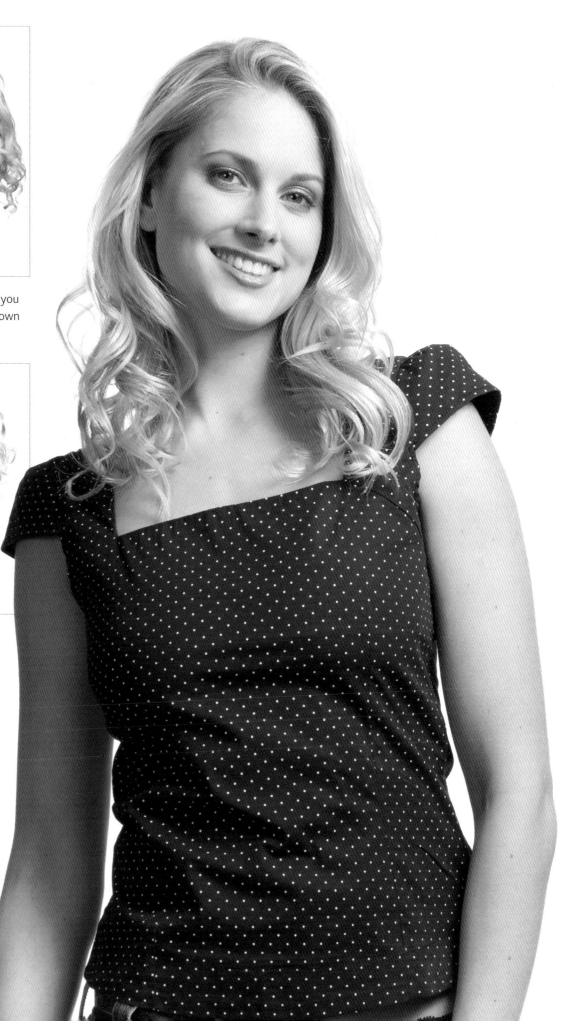

Using tongs to create random spiral curls

You will need
- Heat-protective spray
- Curling tongs
- Hairspray

Rather than creating an all-over curl, tong individual sections of hair then wrap the curled hair around pieces of loose, straighter hair. This is a different take on a classic look and is a great way of ringing the changes!

Stylist's note

Tongs come in different-size barrels, so the shorter the hair, the smaller the barrel-size of tong you need to use.

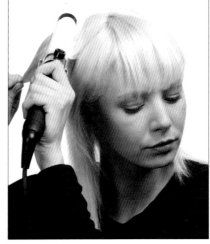

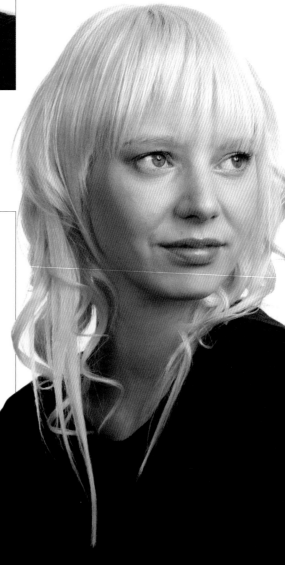

1 Comb through clean, dry hair so that it is tangle-free. Spritz your hair all over with a heat-protective spray to prevent it from scorching or drying out your hair.

2 Taking a small section of hair, place the tongs near the root and clamp shut.

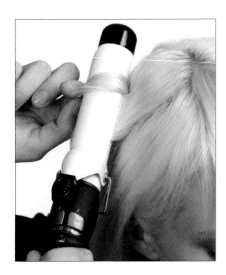

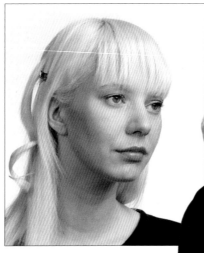

3 Wind the section of hair round the barrel of the tong, working down to the end. Winding this way adds volume and shape.

4 Work random sections of hair in the same way. Finished spirals can be wound around a straight section of hair. Spritz with hairspray for hold.

Using tongs to create all-over curl

A fabulous head of curls is so striking and elegant and makes hair look thicker and more luxurious. Tonging hair will bring out the layers and shape already cut into the hair and, if styled and finished carefully, will stay in as long as needed.

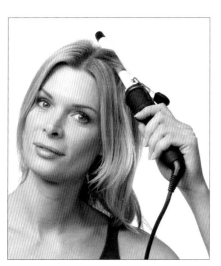

1 Comb dry hair to be tangle-free then spritz all over with a heat-protective spray to prevent it from scorching.

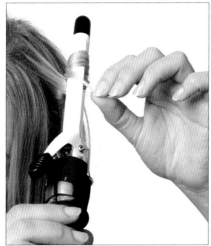

2 Working a small section of hair at a time, place the hot curling tongs in your hair near the roots and wind the hair around the tongs from root to end.

Stylist's note

Taking small sections of hair at a time and ensuring the tongs are always well-heated helps achieve an even curl.

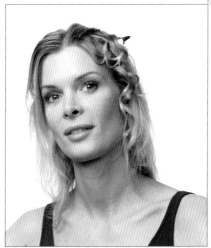

3 Hold the tongs closed for several seconds, allowing the heat to penetrate and set curl into the hair.

4 Continue to tong all the hair in the same way. Allow curls to cool before loosening with your fingers. Spritz with hairspray to hold.

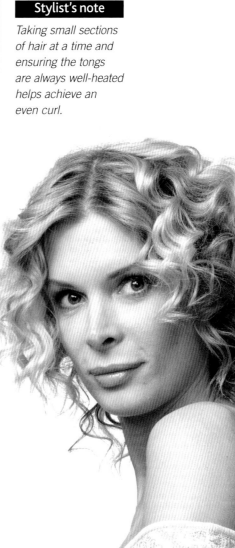

Using irons to create striking blades in shorter hair

This strong look is great fun for girls who dare to be different. It takes time to achieve but will last well throughout the day or evening. The added zig-zag texture keeps it individual and prevents the look becoming too futuristic.

You will need
- Hairbrush
- Strong-hold hairspray
- Straightening irons
- Open-ended pins

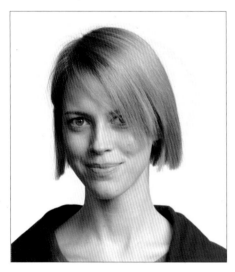

1 Brush clean, dry hair to be completely tangle-free.

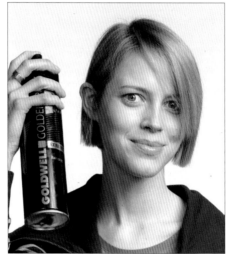

2 Spritz your hair generously all over with a strong-hold hairspray.

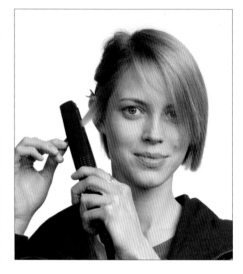

3 Working with very small sections of hair at a time, place the straightening irons near the root, clamp shut and draw through the hair from root to end. Repeat with all your hair.

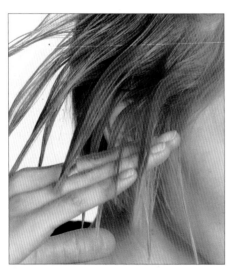

4 Straightened sections must not be brushed or combed, as this would make them separate. Allow them to cool as individual mini blades of hair.

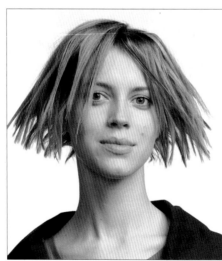

5 Work the whole head in the same way until all hair has been styled into blades.

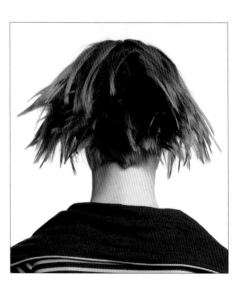

6 Your hair should look like this from the back when you have finished.

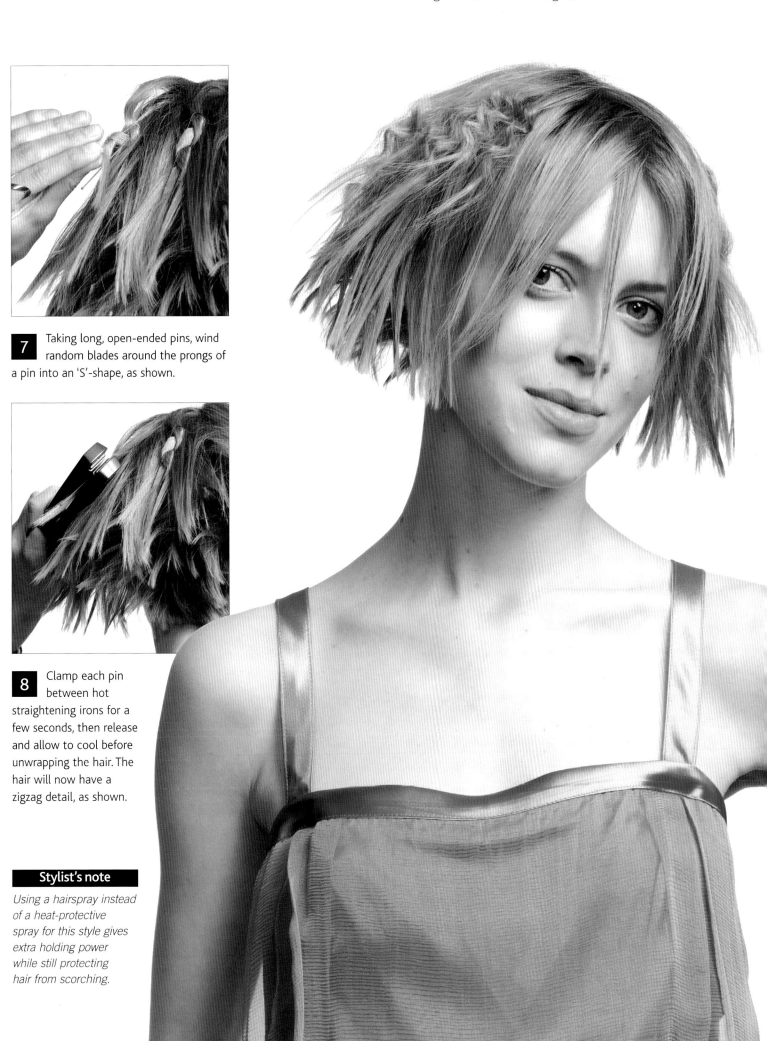

7 Taking long, open-ended pins, wind random blades around the prongs of a pin into an 'S'-shape, as shown.

8 Clamp each pin between hot straightening irons for a few seconds, then release and allow to cool before unwrapping the hair. The hair will now have a zigzag detail, as shown.

Stylist's note

Using a hairspray instead of a heat-protective spray for this style gives extra holding power while still protecting hair from scorching.

Using irons to create movement in shorter hair

Hot straightening irons can be used in many ways, not just to smooth but also to wave hair or to add volume and create movement. It's fun to try different-sized irons, and irons with half-round plates to achieve different finished effects.

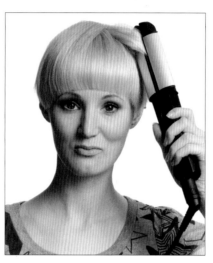

Stylist's note

Some irons have more of a barrel shape, which is useful for creating movement and a more textured finish.

1 Comb dry hair to be tangle-free then spritz all over with a heat-protective spray to prevent it from scorching.

2 Taking a small section of hair, place the straightening irons near the root, clamp shut and draw through the hair, turning the irons slightly to create a bend in the hair.

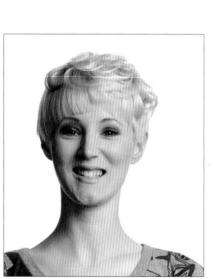

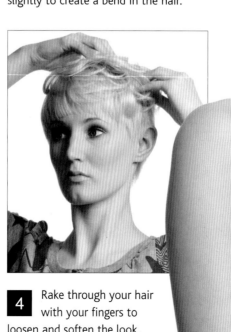

3 Continue applying the irons around the head, working all the hair that is long enough to be shaped in the same way.

4 Rake through your hair with your fingers to loosen and soften the look. Shape as desired and spritz with hairspray to finish.

Using irons to create flicks in layered or graduated hair

Short or mid-length hair looks great when straightening irons are applied to add flicks, kicks and waves, as these can make hair look thicker and more lustrous. For shorter hair, use straightening irons with smaller plates as they are easier to apply.

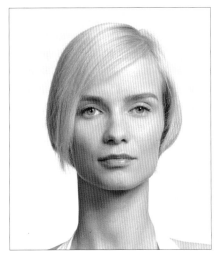

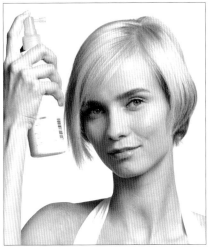

Stylist's note

It's very important to invest in a pair of irons with an automatic cut-off switch and a heat-resistant mat to stand them on.

1 Comb through clean, dry hair to be tangle-free.

2 Spritz heat-protective spray throughout your hair to prevent it from scorching when you apply the straightening irons.

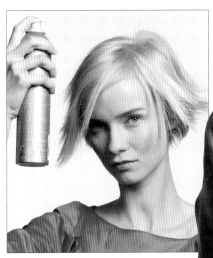

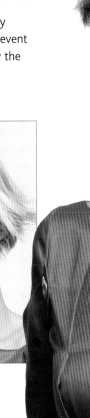

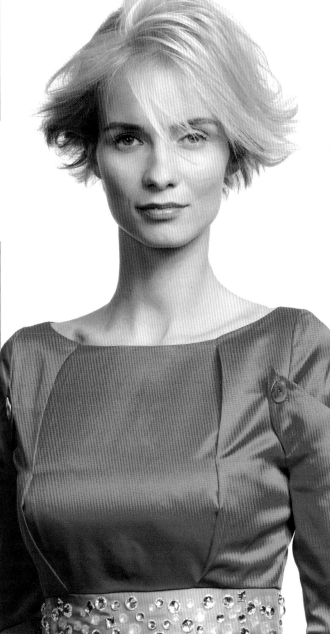

3 Taking a small section of hair, place the straightening irons near the root, clamp shut and draw through the hair, flicking out the wrist on reaching the ends. Repeat with all the hair.

4 Spritz your hair with flexible working spray to finish.

Using irons to straighten hair for a super-sleek look

For a timeless finish that exudes sleek chic, apply straightening irons to dry hair. This is an easy way to get fabulous results, especially on one-length hair, but is a technique that can also add smooth, glossy shine to more layered cuts.

You will need
- Hairbrush
- Sectioning clips
- Heat-protective spray
- Comb
- Straightening irons
- Shine spray

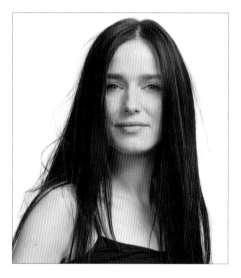

1 Brush clean, dry hair to be completely tangle-free.

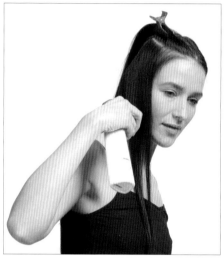

2 Using sectioning clips, divide your hair into manageable sections and spritz all over with a heat-protective spray.

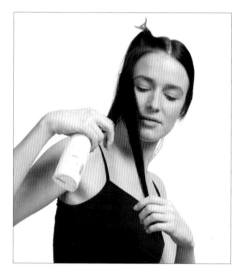

3 Starting at one side, take a small section of hair, comb it through thoroughly and respray it with the heat-protective spray.

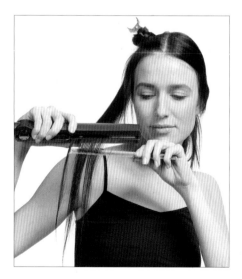

4 Place the straightening irons near the roots, clamp shut and draw through the hair, drawing a comb through in front of the irons.

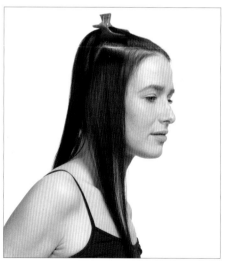

5 The ironed hair should lie flat and smooth, as shown.

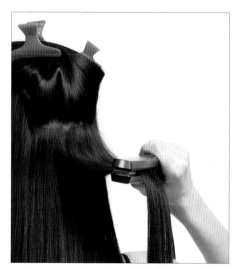

6 Working around the head, apply straightening irons to all sections in the same way.

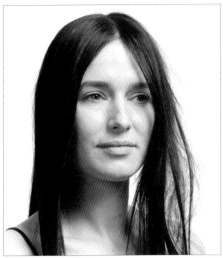

7 This picture shows the contrast between hair that has been ironed and hair that has not.

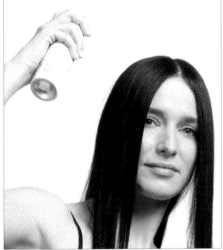

8 When all the hair is ironed, spritz all over with shine spray to finish.

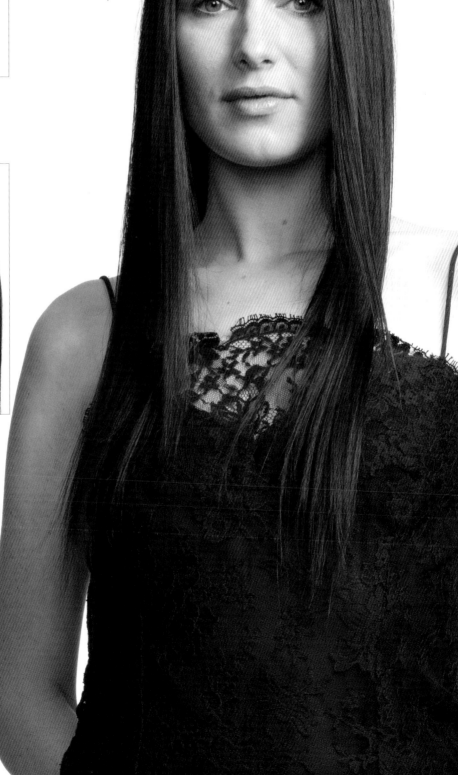

Stylist's note

Use a heat-protective spray after drying and before straightening to help keep hair healthy.

Using irons to create movement in longer hair

It's fun to accentuate the layers and longer length of hair by applying straightening irons in such a way as to add waves and movement. It's also a great way for making hair appear thicker and is less severe than poker-straight hair.

You will need
- Wide-tooth comb
- Styling lotion
- Sectioning clips
- Hairbrush
- Hairdryer
- Hairdryer
- Straightening irons
- Hairspray

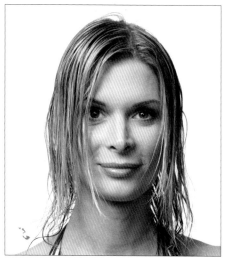

1 Wash your hair, then towel-dry it to be damp rather than wet. Comb through to detangle using a wide-tooth comb, which won't stretch and break your hair.

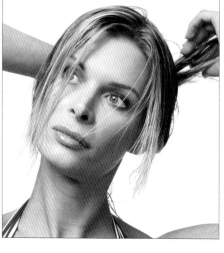

2 Rub a styling product or lotion through your hair so it will retain its shape better when it is dry.

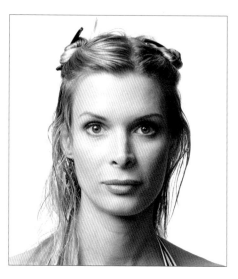

3 Section off the top area of your hair with sectioning clips.

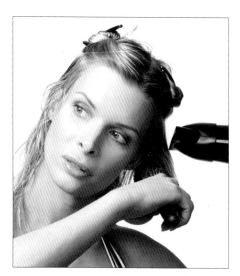

4 Starting with the lower layers, take one small section of hair at a time, wrap it around a brush and blow-dry to give a smooth finish.

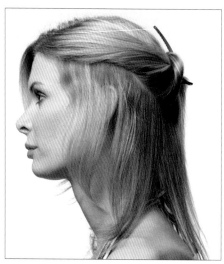

5 When all your hair is completely dry, section off the top area again and clip it out of the way.

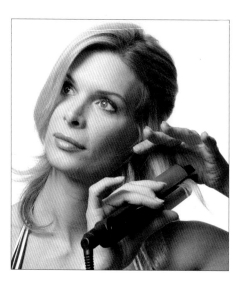

6 Taking a small section of hair from underneath, place the straightening irons near the root, clamp shut and draw through the hair, flicking the ends out.

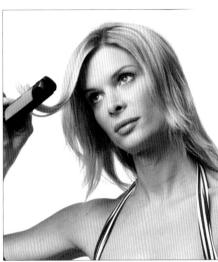

7 Continue around your head and through the top section until all of your hair is flicked out at the ends.

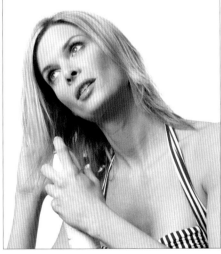

8 Spritz your hair with a light to medium-hold spray, focusing on spritzing the ends from underneath to encourage the kick.

Stylist's note

It's important to blow-dry hair properly before applying irons to create the movement or the style will drop quickly.

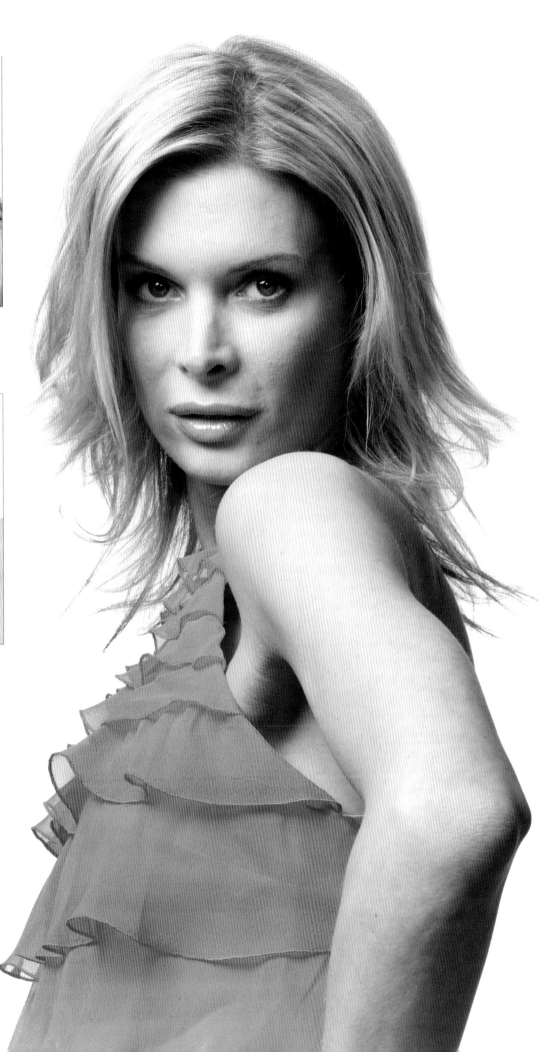

Crimping loose hair for all-over texture

You will need
- Comb or hairbrush
- Heat-protective spray
- Sectioning clips
- Crimping irons
- Hairspray

Crimping your hair is always a fantastic way to really plump up fine or flat hair or add texture and volume for when you want to wear your hair up. The secret is to not crimp too close to the roots or your style will balloon!

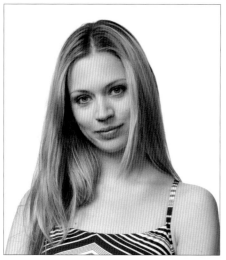

1 Brush dry hair to be completely tangle-free and smooth.

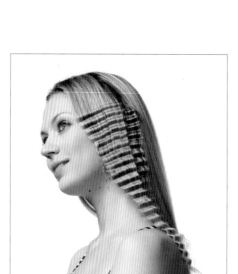

2 Spritz your hair all over with a heat-protective spray to prevent it from scorching or drying out your hair.

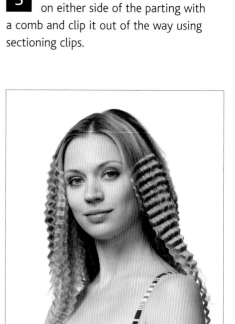

3 Section off the top area of hair on either side of the parting with a comb and clip it out of the way using sectioning clips.

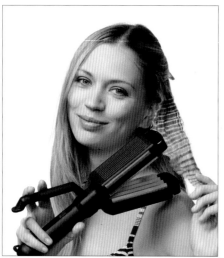

4 Starting with the underneath section, apply hot crimping irons to one small section at a time. Hold closed for 3 seconds. Repeat, working down the length of the hair.

5 Work all the underneath hair before moving on to the top section. Ensure crimps are placed evenly or the result will look odd.

6 Crimped hair should look like this when you have finished.

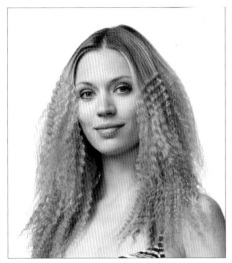

7 Loosen the crimps by running your fingers through your hair.

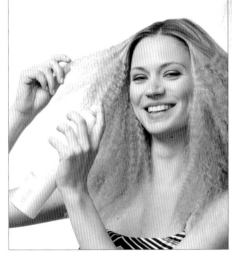

8 Tease sections of hair to create volume and a softer, more angel-hair finish. Spray with hairspray to hold.

Stylist's note

Remember to carefully position the irons to form an even crimp pattern down each length of hair.

Crimping dressed hair for partial texture

You can have fun and add crimps to your hair without committing to an all-over crimped finish. Decide first how to dress your finished hair to show off the textured areas, then select sections of hair to crimp, creating a style that works for you.

You will need
- Comb
- Hairband (headband)
- Heat-protective spray
- Crimping irons

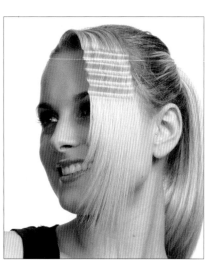

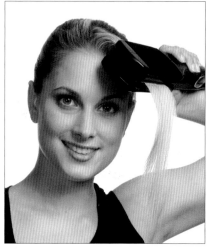

Stylist's note

If you have fine hair, be careful not to hold the crimping irons closed for too long or you risk scorching your hair. Ensure you always apply heat-protective spray before using crimping irons.

1 Comb dry hair smooth. Secure in a ponytail at the back of the head with a hairband (headband), leaving some front hair free. Spritz loose hair with heat-protective spray

2 Starting with the loose front section, clamp the crimping irons on the chosen area – starting near the top but not too near the root. Hold for a few seconds.

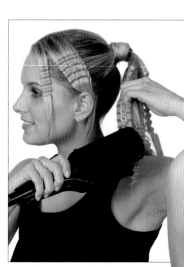

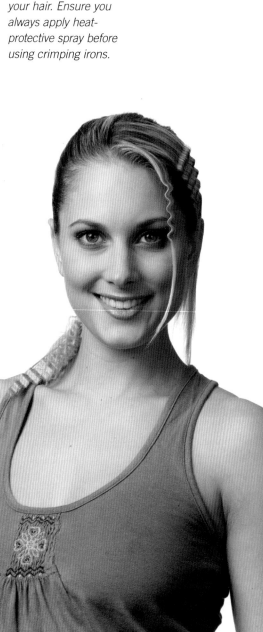

3 Release the irons but do not brush your hair as this will cause the crimped area to frizz. Leave hair to cool.

4 Select random sections of the ponytail, spritz with heat-protective spray and repeat the crimping action.

Crimping loose hair for a random texture effect

For a loose, fresh style that is easy to achieve, crimp random sections of hair as shown opposite, but leave it to hang loose. This technique works well on mid-length to longer hair, adding interest without too much volume.

Stylist's note

Crimping shorter hair can add too much width, which is very hard to balance in a style, so it is advisable to use crimps only if you have mid-length or longer hair.

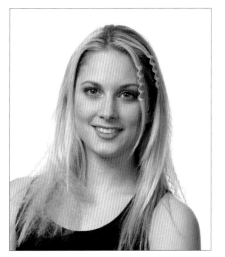

1 Follow the technique shown opposite up to Step 3, then remove the hairband (headband). Shake your hair free but do not brush it.

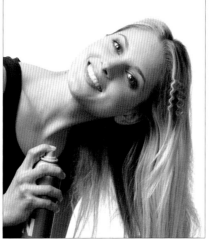

2 Generously spritz your hair all over with a light-hold spray to add more volume and to ensure the style will hold.

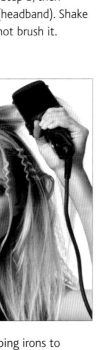

3 Apply the crimping irons to random sections of hair that have not yet been worked, especially at the top and back of the head, and hold for a few seconds.

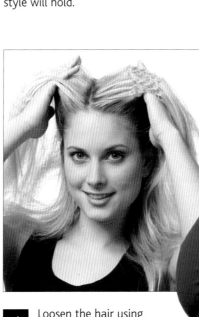

4 Loosen the hair using your fingers to break up the crimped sections slightly and to add extra volume and movement to the style.

Setting hair on heated rollers

Using heated rollers means you can multi-task while getting ready! The hair can be set on rollers and you can then move around and continue dressing and applying make-up until the rollers have cooled and are ready for removing.

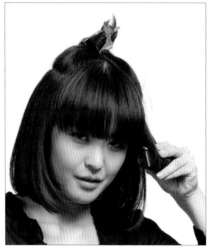

Stylist's note

A set of heated rollers will include a variety of different-sized rollers. Put larger ones through the top sections to create lift and movement.

1 Plug in the heated rollers. Apply styling lotion liberally to dry, detangled hair. Section off the top-back area and start working the lower and front areas of hair first.

2 Taking small sections of hair from these lower and front areas, wind the pre-heated rollers from end to root and use pins to hold them in place.

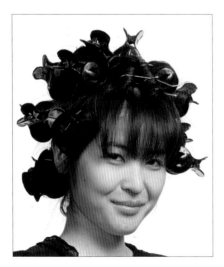

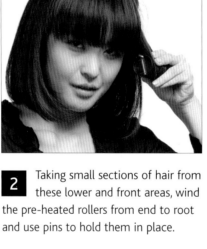

3 Working through all the hair, including the sectioned-off top section, wrap all your hair in rollers and leave to cool completely – about 30 minutes.

4 Remove the rollers and loosen the curls using your fingers. Pin up random sections to create an individual style. Spritz with hairspray.

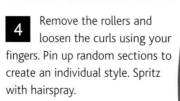

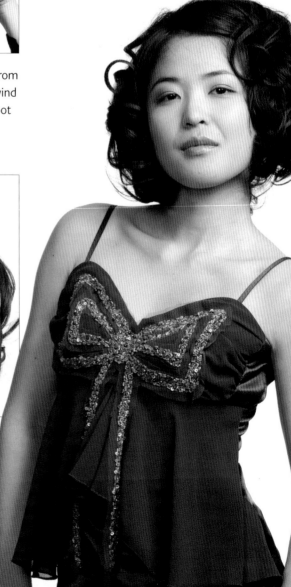

Setting hair on self-gripping rollers

For a softer set or for when heated rollers are not an option, use rollers that stay in all on their own. Lightweight and available in different sizes, they are perfect for hair that curls quickly and easily, and they are comfortable to use, too.

Stylist's note

Self-gripping rollers are a fantastic way of curling hair when you are on holiday as they are easy and light to pack and don't need to be heated.

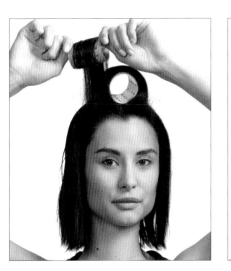

1 Wash your hair, then towel-dry it to be damp rather than wet. Comb through to detangle using a wide-tooth comb, which won't stretch and break your hair.

2 Spritz your hair all over with styling lotion to help set and hold the style.

3 Taking one small section of hair at a time and starting at the top of your head, wrap hair around the rollers, working from the end to the root. Repeat with all your hair.

4 Allow hair to dry naturally (or apply a gentle heat using a hairdryer). Remove the rollers, loosen your hair with your fingers and spray to hold.

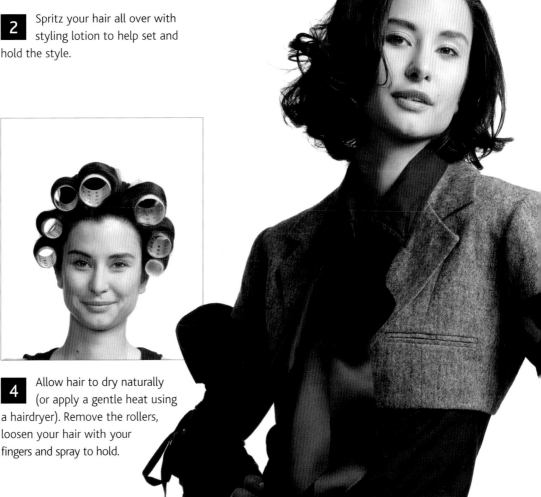

Using bendable rods to create an even curl

Using long fabric or plastic bendable rods is a great way to create even, tight curls. Wound into damp hair, they can then be left to dry naturally. This is a gentle curling technique that is ideal for more fragile colour-treated or even permed hair.

You will need
- Wide-tooth comb
- Light gel-based product
- Sectioning clips
- Bendable rods
- Hairdryer
- Finishing spray
- Pins

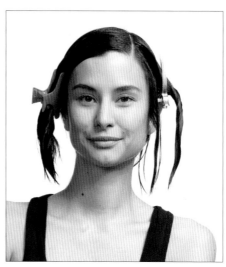

1 Wash your hair, then towel-dry it to be just damp. Comb through to detangle using a wide-tooth comb. Apply a light gel-based styling product and work through the hair from root to end.

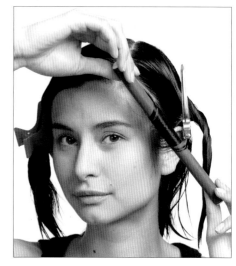

2 Section your hair into manageable working sections using sectioning clips, twisting the hair and clipping it out of the way so that it doesn't dry out while you are positioning the rods.

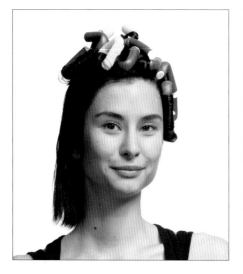

3 Taking a small section of hair, place a rod near the end and wind up to the roots. Bend the ends of the rod inwards to hold it in place.

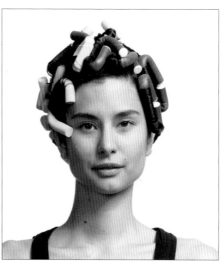

4 Repeat the technique and place rods all around the head, working section by section.

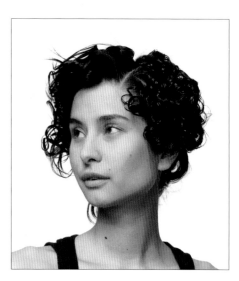

5 When all the hair is wound and all the rods are bent into position, your head should look like this. Allow hair to dry naturally.

6 Remove the rods by unbending them and gently pulling them out, working systematically through the hair.

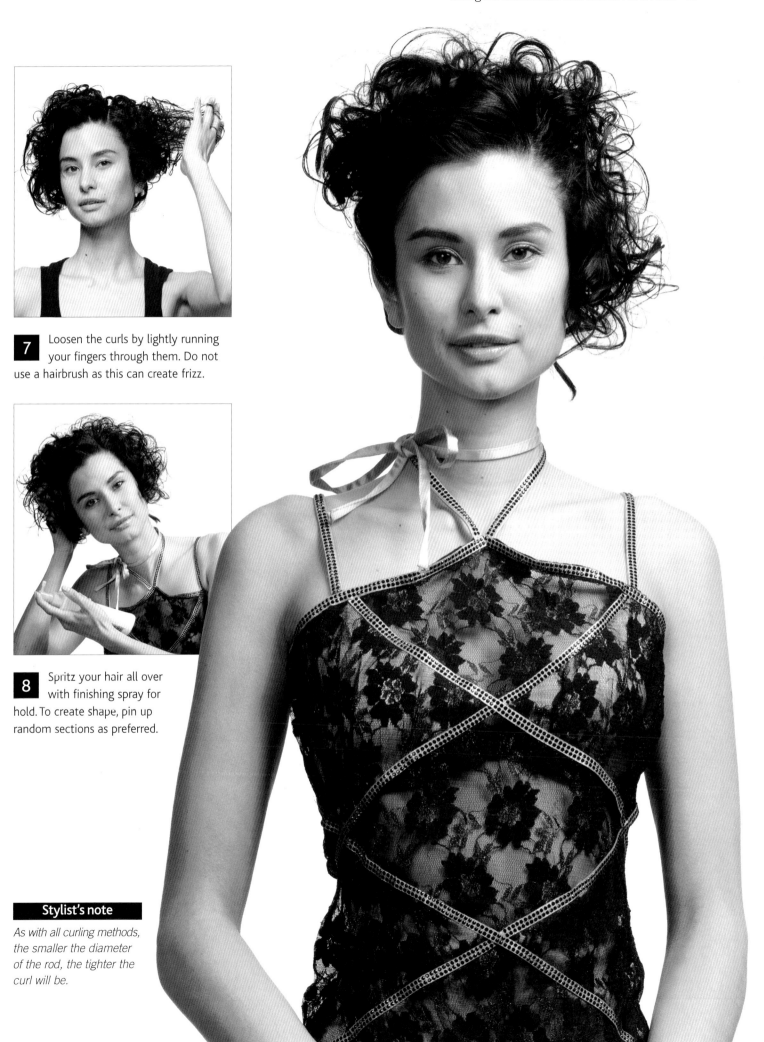

7 Loosen the curls by lightly running your fingers through them. Do not use a hairbrush as this can create frizz.

8 Spritz your hair all over with finishing spray for hold. To create shape, pin up random sections as preferred.

Stylist's note

As with all curling methods, the smaller the diameter of the rod, the tighter the curl will be.

Using pin curls to create a gentle, tumbling curl

This is a handy technique for creating curls overnight as pin curls are much more comfortable to sleep in than rollers. It is also perfect for when you are on the move as a pack of pins takes up very little room in a suitcase.

You will need
- Wide-tooth comb
- Styling lotion
- Hairgrips (bobby pins)
- Hairdryer

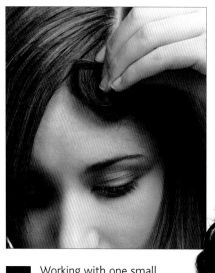

Stylist's note

The smaller the sections of hair pinned in place and the longer they are left in to set, the curlier the finished look will be.

1 Comb dry hair to be tangle-free and spritz all over with a styling lotion to help hold the curl.

2 Working with one small section at a time, wrap pieces of hair round your fingers, as though winding on a roller, to form a curl shape.

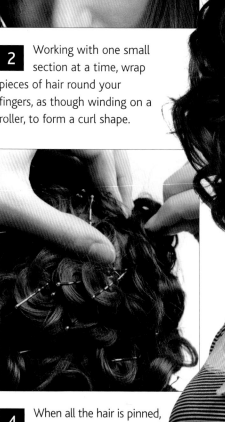

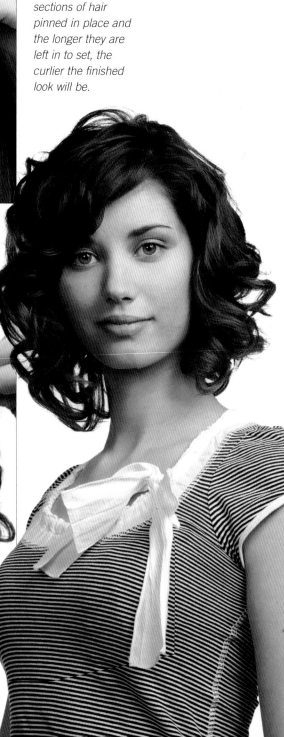

3 Lay the curl flat against your head and grip it in place with one pin, or two pins crossed if you require extra hold.

4 When all the hair is pinned, apply heat or leave overnight. Remove the pins and finger-comb your hair, then style.

Using barrel curls to create volume and soft curl

For a look that's reminiscent of a natural wave or curl and which looks just as glamorous and stylish, practise this simple technique for barrel curls. It produces a gentle, soft, cascading curl effect.

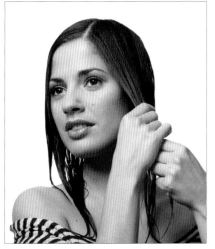

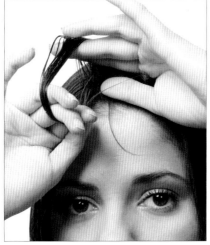

Stylist's note

To speed up the set, dry hair with a hairdryer but use a low heat-setting to avoid blasting the barrel curls out of shape.

1 Wash your hair, then towel-dry it to be damp rather than wet. Comb through to detangle using a wide-tooth comb. Apply styling lotion generously throughout the hair.

2 Taking a small section of hair at a time, wrap the hair loosely round your fingers to create a barrel shape, or large loop.

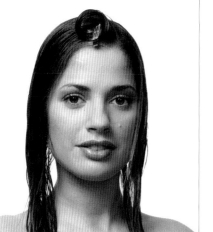

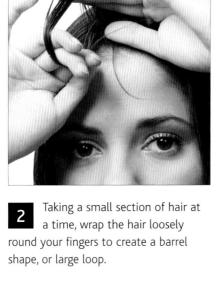

3 Use a hairgrip (bobby pin) or clip to secure the curl to your head, as shown, then continue to work the remaining hair into curls in the same way.

4 Allow your hair to dry. Remove the hairgrips and loosen the curl using your fingers or by brushing. Spritz with a shine spray.

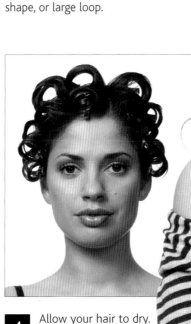

Using plaits to create a gentle wave

By simply braiding hair into plaits and leaving it for a few hours, you can add a great-looking gentle wave and movement into any hair type. It's a handy method that can be adapted for keeping hair tidy then later revealing a great style.

You will need
- Hairbrush
- Sectioning clips
- Hairspray
- Hairbands (headbands)
- Shine spray

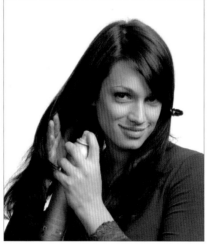

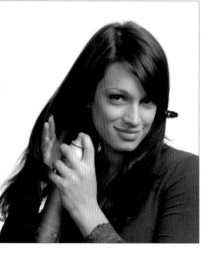

Stylist's note

The tighter you weave the plaits, the more pronounced the wave will be.

1 Brush dry hair until it is smooth and tangle-free.

2 Section your hair down the centre back of the head. Clip one half out of the way, then liberally spritz loose hair with hairspray for hold.

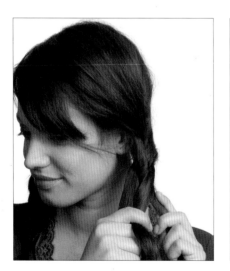

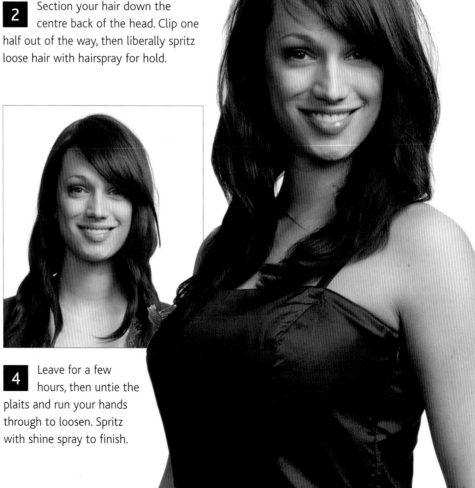

3 Divide this loose hair into three equal strands and weave them into a loose plait (braid), securing the end with a hairband (headband). Repeat on the other side.

4 Leave for a few hours, then untie the plaits and run your hands through to loosen. Spritz with shine spray to finish.

Using multi-plaits to create a stonger wave

Braiding hair into several plaits will accentuate any natural wave in the hair. You can decide how many plaits you need, depending on how thick your hair is. However many you need, make sure they are similar-sized for an even finish.

You will need
- Comb
- Styling lotion
- Sectioning clips
- Hairbands (headbands)
- Hairdryer
- Hairspray

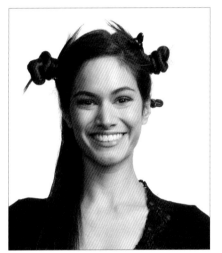

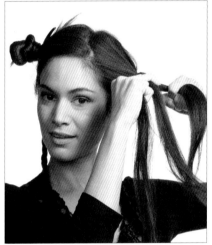

Stylist's note

Starting with damp hair and leaving hair to dry overnight gives a more distinctly textured effect.

1 Comb through damp hair. Apply styling lotion throughout, then section your hair into a minimum of four similar-sized sections. Make more if you want a more textured finish.

2 Work through each section in turn, weaving the hair into plaits (braids) and securing the ends with hairbands (headbands).

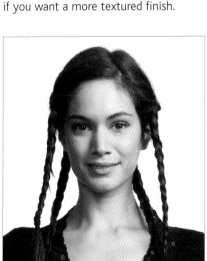

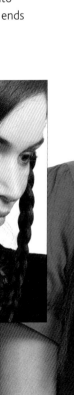

3 When you have finished braiding the hair, apply heat from a hairdryer for speed or leave hair to dry naturally – this will probably take at least 2 hours.

4 When the plaits are dry, remove them and run your hands through the hair to loosen. Style as you like and spray for hold.

Forming a Marcel wave for a retro look

For a retro look use this very old technique, which creates a stylized wave in the hair. It's effective placed throughout the front section to emulate the 'screen sirens' of old. It will take practice to perfect but is well worth the effort.

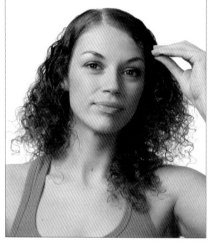

1 Wash your hair, then blow-dry it to be completely dry.

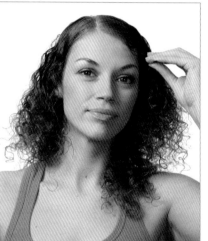

2 Apply a liquid gel or strong-hold styling product through the top sections of your hair (from the top of your head to ear level), then comb this area smooth.

Stylist's note

For this wave, use flat metal clips, which will hold the hair without leaving an unsightly ridge in the dry hair.

3 Use your fingers to smooth and hold hair from the hairline down, then push the lower hair back up towards the root, creating an 'S'-bend. Hold with a clip.

4 Form a second wave below the first and grip in place. Repeat on the other side. Leave to set, then remove the clips.

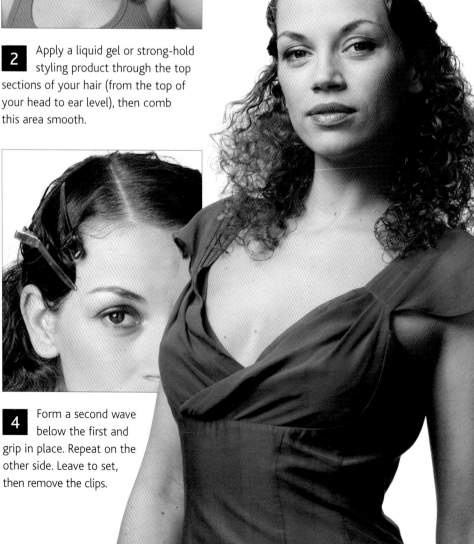

Using your fingers to shape shorter hair

You can achieve fantastic shape and texture in short hair without spending hours in front of the mirror with a hairdryer. The trick is to apply a texturizing product to hair that is just dry, then work the hair into shape with your fingers.

You will need
- Comb
- Light styling product

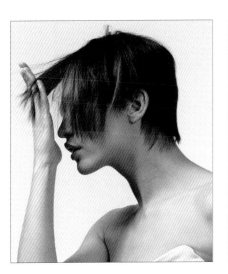

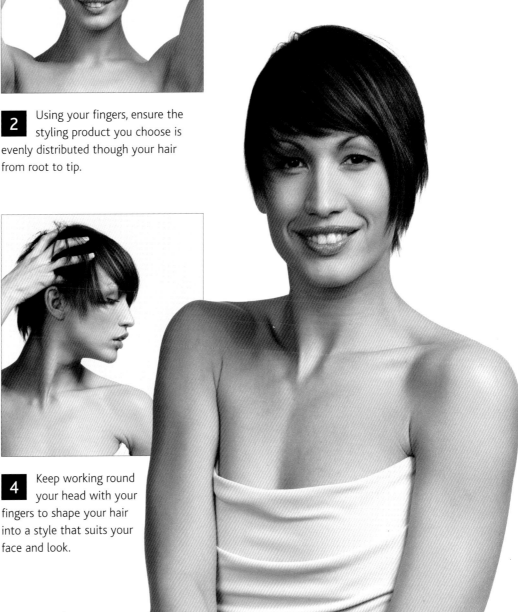

Stylist's note

Choosing the right styling product for your hair type will help you achieve this look. Ask your salon for advice.

1 Wash your hair and towel-dry it lightly. Comb a light-hold gel, spray or lotion styling product through your hair.

2 Using your fingers, ensure the styling product you choose is evenly distributed though your hair from root to tip.

3 Tease the hair into shape using your fingers. Keep lifting it at the roots to add height and to avoid a flat finish.

4 Keep working round your head with your fingers to shape your hair into a style that suits your face and look.

Using gel to create a smooth, wet look on shorter hair

This delightful finish best suits elfin cuts and strong face shapes. It is a great way to accentuate a good head shape and a strong cut. It requires some confidence to wear, but is oh-so-striking. What could be easier?

You will need
- Wide-tooth comb
- Wet-look gel

1 Wash your hair, then towel-dry it to be damp rather than wet. Comb through to detangle using a wide-tooth comb, which won't stretch and break your hair.

2 Squirt some styling gel into the palm of your hand, then rub your hands together.

Stylist's note

Gel is a product with such great staying power that it can be used to sweep fringes (bangs) to one side and they'll stay put.

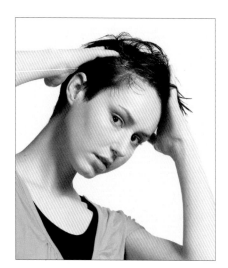

3 Apply the gel to your hair with your fingers, ensuring it is worked through hair from root to tip and is evenly distributed over your head.

4 Comb your hair into the style of your choice and leave to dry.

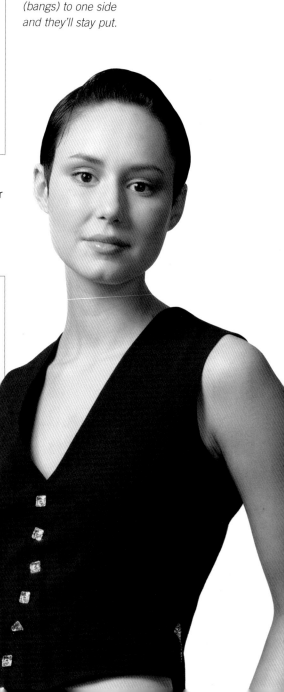

Using gel to create spikes on shorter hair

You will need
- Wide-tooth comb
- Gel
- Hairdryer
- Comb

If hair is cut in layers with a mixture of short and long lengths then it is ideal for this look, which makes a striking change from flat or multi-textured short looks. The shorter layers help the longer lengths to stand up more.

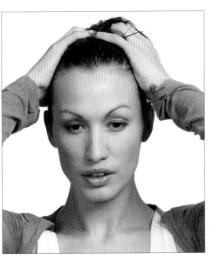

Stylist's note

Gel is available in strong, medium and light-hold formulas, so be sure to select one that is right for your hair type.

1 Wash your hair, then towel-dry it to be damp rather than wet. Comb through to detangle using a wide-tooth comb, which won't stretch and break your hair.

2 Apply gel by tipping the product into the palm of your hand, then working it through the hair, using the fingers to ensure it is distributed from root to tip.

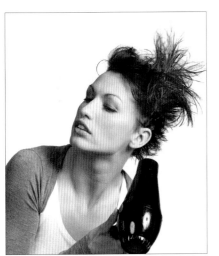

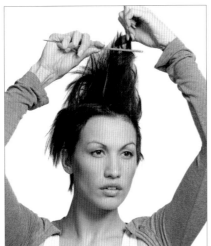

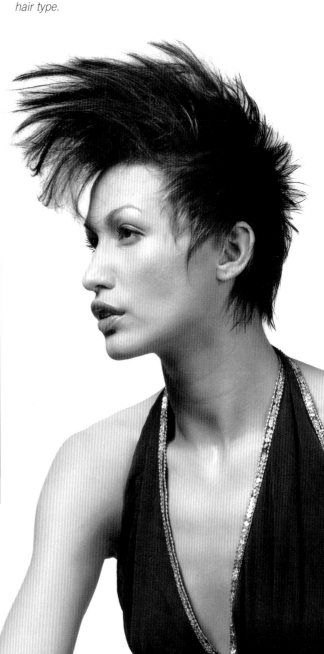

3 Blast-dry your hair with the hairdryer, paying particular attention to the roots to create lift. Direct the airflow to blow from underneath to add volume.

4 Twist random sections of hair, then backcomb these for added height where required and to create defined shape.

Using mousse to create a bedhead finish on longer hair

Work with product to build up texture and volume in your hair, creating a look that is vibrant and youthful. This is a great way to prevent longer hair looking drab or dull and it makes heavier, thicker hair look full of life instead of falling flat.

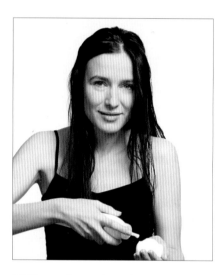

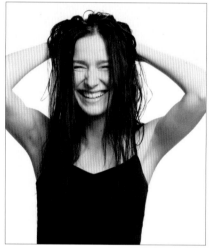

Stylist's note

When rough-drying hair, run your fingers through the hair frequently to prevent tangles forming.

1 Wash your hair, then towel-dry it to be damp. Comb through to detangle using a wide-tooth comb. Squirt some mousse into the palm of your hand.

2 Rub your hands together, then work the volumizing mousse into your hair from root to tip using your fingers to distribute it evenly.

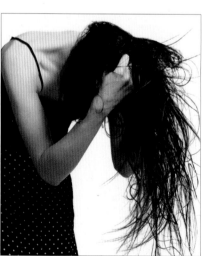

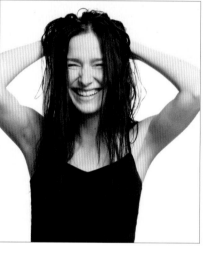

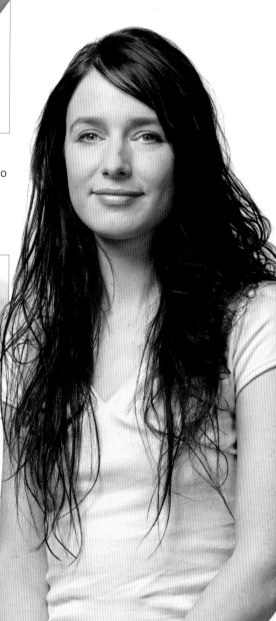

3 Tip your head upside-down and scrunch your hair up from the lengths to the roots. Leave hair to dry naturally, scrunching your hair again if necessary to add texture.

4 To finish, spritz hair all over with a texturizing spray to enhance the movement and texture you have created.

Fitting and wearing a wig with a natural hair fringe

You will need
- Comb
- Hairnet (optional)
- Wig
- Hairbrush

Blend a wig with your natural hair to disguise problems such as colour regrowth at the roots, conceal ultra-fine hair or to add length. Leaving your fringe free will make the look more natural, but only if you make a good colour match.

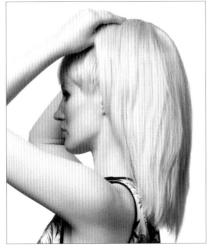

Stylist's note

It's important to place the wig on your head from back to front, keeping your natural fringe lying flat.

1 Comb dry hair to be as smooth and flat as possible. Tuck longer hair into a hairnet to keep it as close and flat to the head as possible.

2 Position the wig on the crown of your head, ready to put on from back to front.

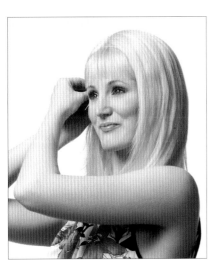

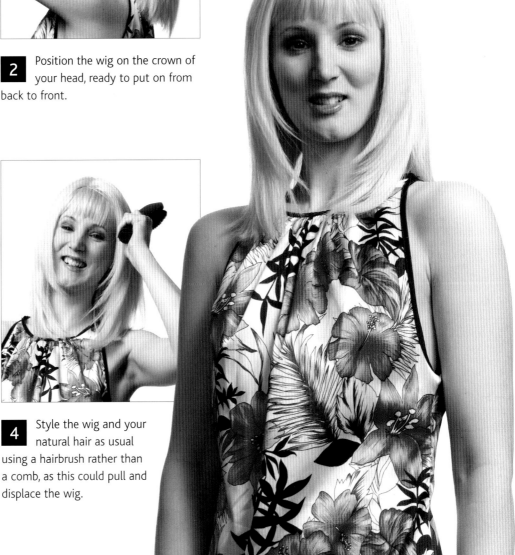

3 Draw the wig forward into place, leaving the fringe (bangs) free, and fix the wig in place using its own inbuilt combs.

4 Style the wig and your natural hair as usual using a hairbrush rather than a comb, as this could pull and displace the wig.

Fitting and wearing a whole-head wig

Ring the changes by wearing a wig! You can alter your hair colour, length and texture in an instant. There is a huge range of wigs available, and modern wigs are light, comfortable and look very natural if they are worn properly.

1 Brush dry hair to be smooth and spritz all over with hairspray to keep hair in place.

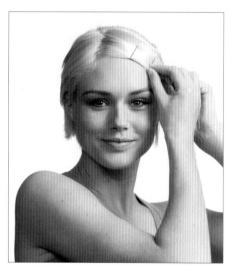

2 Long hair should be tied up at the back with a hairband (headband). Grip a fringe (bangs) out of the way with hairgrips (bobby pins), to keep the hairline as clean as possible.

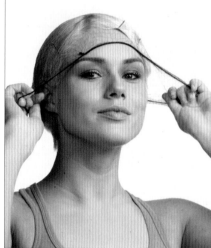

3 Place a hairnet over your head to keep hair as flat and as close to the head as possible.

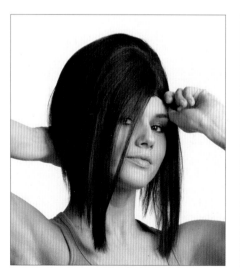

4 Place the wig on to your head, taking care to fit it from front to back and matching up the front edge of the wig base to the front hairline.

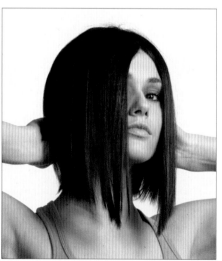

5 Pull the back of the wig base down to the base of your head so it's a snug fit.

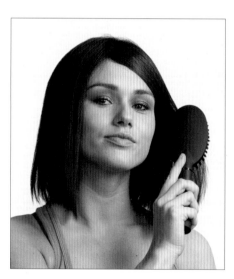

6 Once the wig is in place it should feel comfortable and match your hairline. Now you can style the hair as usual. Brush smooth.

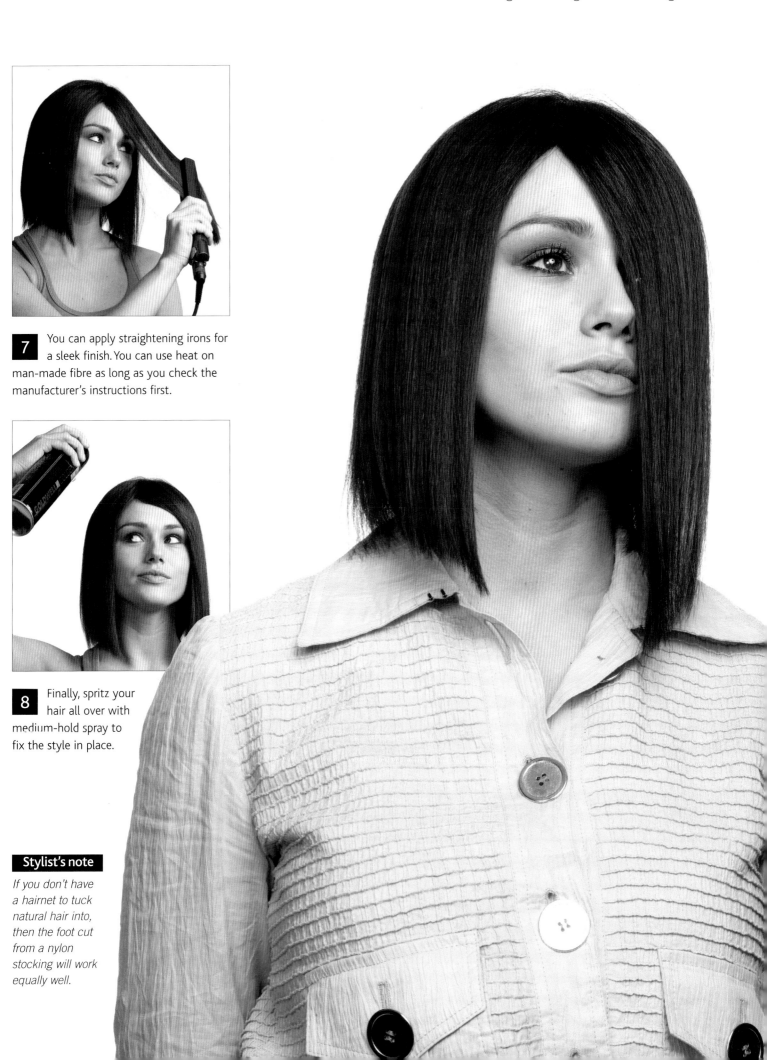

7 You can apply straightening irons for a sleek finish. You can use heat on man-made fibre as long as you check the manufacturer's instructions first.

8 Finally, spritz your hair all over with medium-hold spray to fix the style in place.

Stylist's note

If you don't have a hairnet to tuck natural hair into, then the foot cut from a nylon stocking will work equally well.

Fitting and wearing a hair weft

Use clip-in, narrow wefts of false hair as a quick and fun way to jazz up your hair colour. Just pick the colour you want, clip it in and go. When you've had enough, they are simple to remove and can be reused countless times.

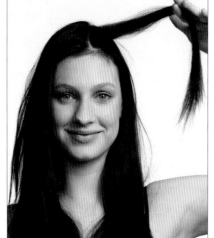

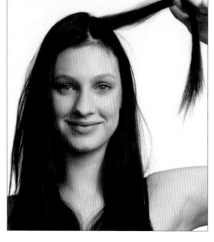

Stylist's note

Placing the weft just below the line of your parting makes it easier to disguise the join and blend it in with your hair.

1 Brush dry hair to be smooth and tangle-free.

2 Take a section of hair from just below the natural parting and lift it back and out of the way (in effect creating a temporary second parting). Secure with a sectioning clip.

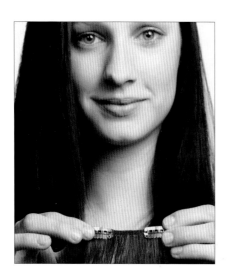

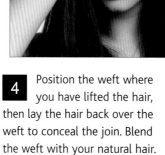

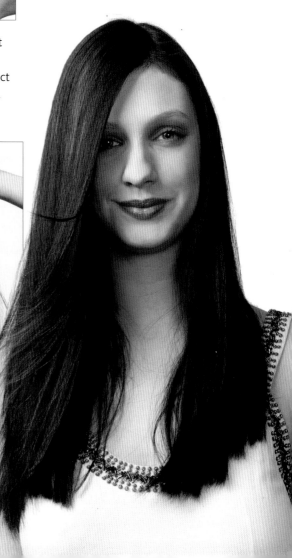

3 Pick up the weft and hold it at the top so that the integral combs face down. Depending on the width of the weft there may be two or more integral combs.

4 Position the weft where you have lifted the hair, then lay the hair back over the weft to conceal the join. Blend the weft with your natural hair.

Fitting and wearing a false fringe

It's so easy to use false hair pieces to quickly change your style. Available with a variety of fixings, from clips to bands and internal grippers, choose between man-made fibre and real hair. Nobody will ever know unless you tell them!

You will need
- Comb
- Light-hold hairspray
- False fringe (bangs) on a band

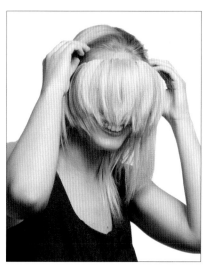

1 Comb dry hair away from your forehead. Apply light-hold hairspray to smooth the hair further. Select a hairpiece that matches your hair colour as closely as possible.

2 The false fringe (bangs) shown here is on a band to hold it in place. Place the fringe on your forehead and position the band to sit behind your ears, as shown here.

Stylist's note

Mixing false and natural hair works best when you are careful to select a great colour match. Ask for a second opinion when choosing as it is easier for someone else to judge.

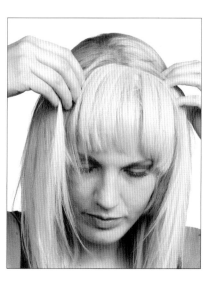

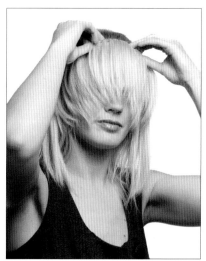

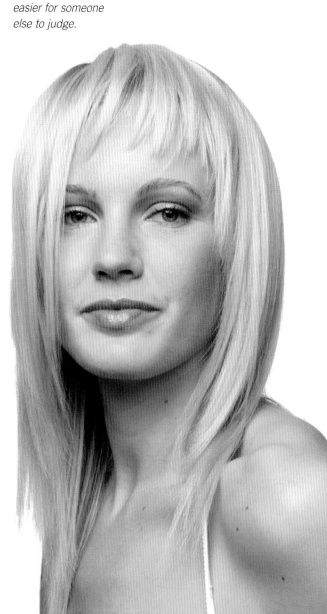

3 Push back the band and draw the fringe up so it sits neatly along your natural hairline. Blend the false hair in with your natural hair.

4 Style all of the hair as usual. You can use heat on man-made fibre as long as you check the manufacturer's instructions first.

Fitting and wearing a false ponytail

To lengthen and fill out a natural ponytail so that it becomes fantastically luxurious and more eye-catching, augment your own hair with a ready-made hairpiece. It's an instant solution and can be very quickly and easily fixed in place.

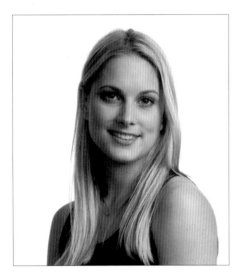

1 Brush dry hair to be neat and tangle-free.

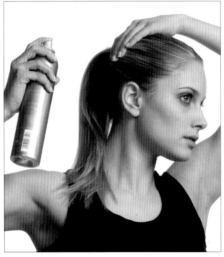

2 Draw your hair into a ponytail, secure with a hairband (headband) and spritz with hairspray. Use the palms of your hands to run over the sides of your head and calm any flyaway hairs.

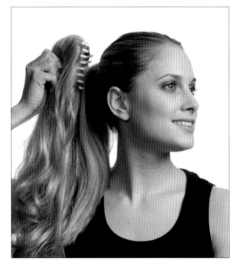

3 Position the false ponytail over the natural one. Select a hairpiece that's a good colour match and which is longer than the natural ponytail.

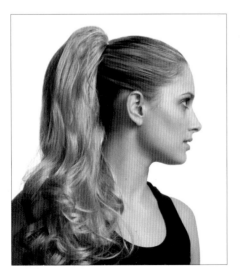

4 This false piece has a crocodile-clip grip mechanism which clasps shut over the base of the natural ponytail.

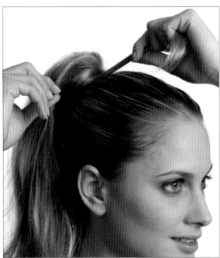

5 Hide the join by wrapping a small section of natural hair around the base of the ponytail and gripping it in place with hairgrips (bobby pins).

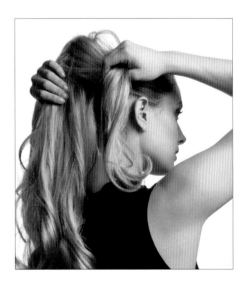

6 Blend the tail of natural and false hair with your fingers.

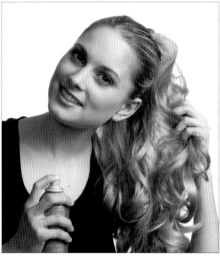

7 Spritz the ponytail all over with shine spray.

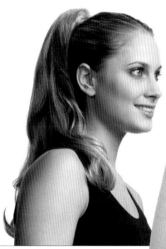

8 You should not be able to see where the false hair is affixed when you have finished; it should look natural.

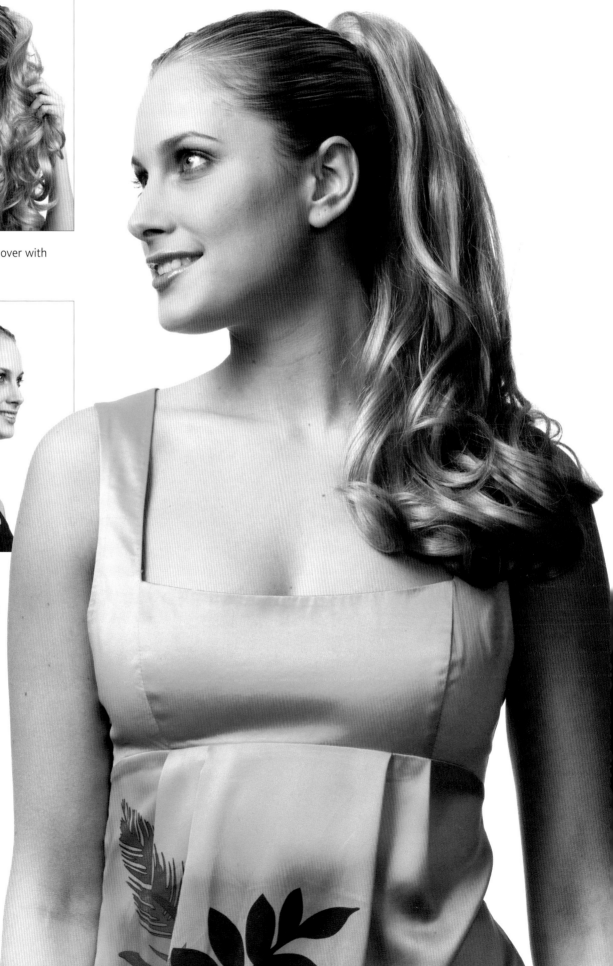

Stylist's note

When adding a curled hairpiece to straight hair, you will need first to curl your own hair in order to blend the hairpiece more convincingly.

A range of fringe finishes for different effects

A fringe is a great face-framing feature of a haircut that can also draw attention to your eyes and bring out the colour and texture of a hairstyle. It's versatile too. Alter the way you wear a fringe and see how it changes your look.

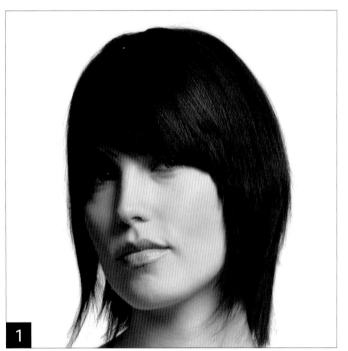

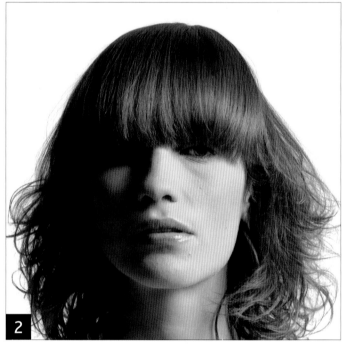

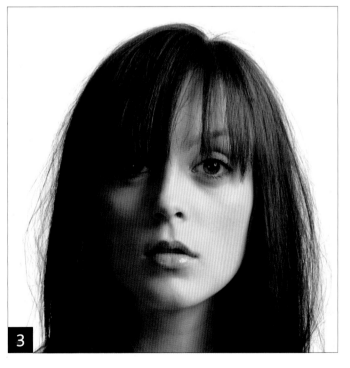

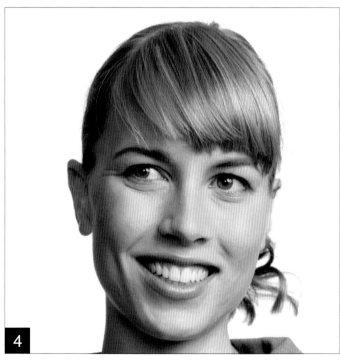

1 Accentuate a strong fringe (bangs) as a feature by blow-drying it smooth and applying a small amount of shine crème. Push the fringe slightly to one side if you like, to soften the look. Super elegant.

2 Eyes peeping out from under a very full fringe can be very seductive. Create this style of fringe by blow-drying it to be ultra-smooth against a textured bob – it's a great dramatic contrast.

3 Opt for a deep fringe on a long style as it keeps the look youthful and fresh. You don't need to wear the fringe all one length – it will be easier to carry off if it is shattered or chopped into slightly.

4 A fringe is a great way to balance a longer, oblong-shaped face and looks great when the rest of the hair is tied back.

5 Moving a parting lower to one side gives the effect of a long fringe worn on one side. Use smoothing crème or spray to keep hair in place.

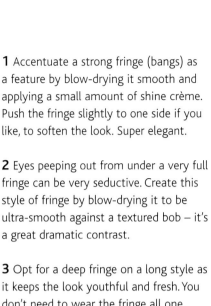

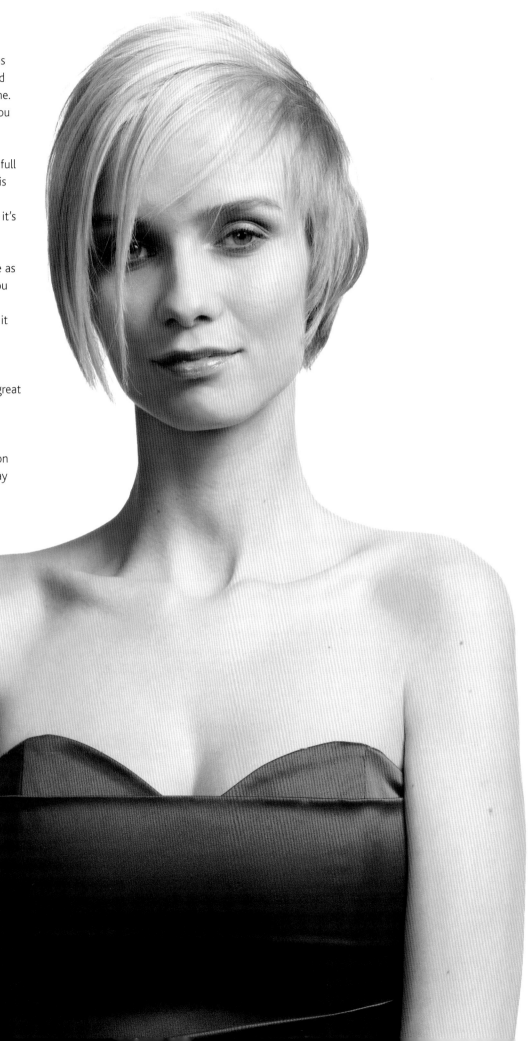

5

Creating a rolling ponytail on mid-length or longer hair

If you don't have the time or enough confidence to put your hair in a full up-do, then this twisted style is perfect as it is easier to do than you think and makes an attractive eye-catching look. Simply roll and go!

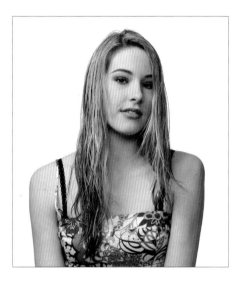

1 Wash your hair, then towel-dry it to be damp rather than wet. Comb through to detangle using a wide-tooth comb, which won't stretch and break your hair.

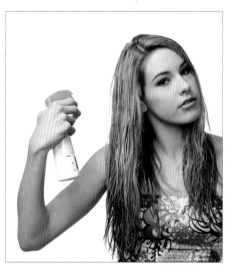

2 Spritz your hair all over with a heat-protective spray to prevent scorching hair when drying it.

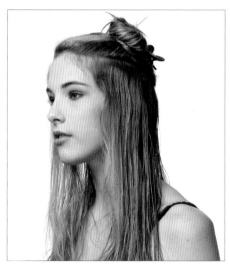

3 Section off the top area using sectioning clips. Position the diffuser under the ends and mid-lengths of your hair and work around your head drying hair in sections, ensuring it rests on the diffuser.

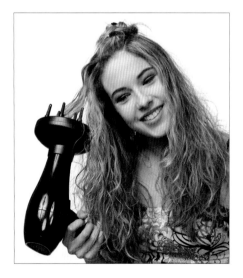

4 Remove the sectioning clips and work through the top section of hair in the same way, until all your hair is completely dry.

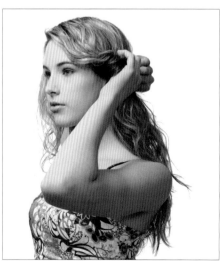

5 Take a panel of hair from the front of the ear at one side and start loosely twisting it towards the back of your head.

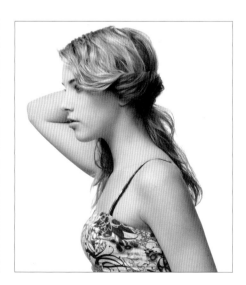

6 Draw in more hair as you work towards the back of your head, keeping fingers open and continuing to loosely twist the hair.

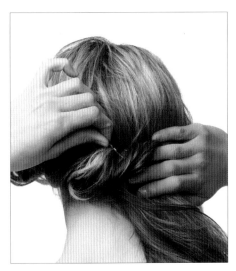

7 Grip the roll of hair to secure to the back of your head at a point just past the centre.

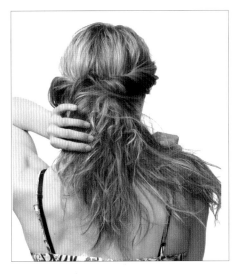

8 Repeat the process, starting at the other side of your head and gripping this second section over the first at the back. Tease the loose ends to blend and to fan out.

Stylist's note

Diffuse-drying the hair before you create the ponytail adds body and shows off the roll detail of this style to better effect.

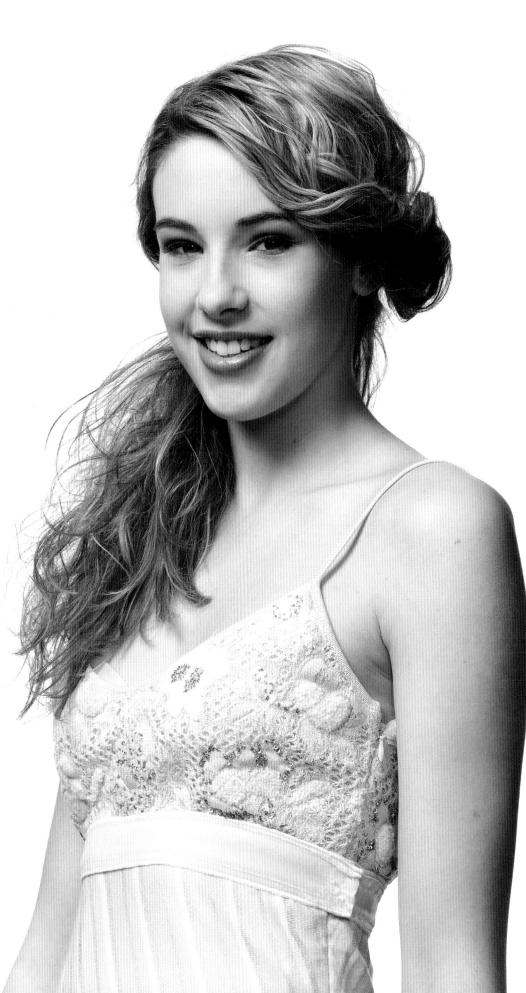

Placing ponytails for different effects

Have you ever wondered how to move on from schoolgirl ponytails to the more sophisticated looks on the fashion pages of magazines or catwalk shows? Perfect placement is the key, so here's the know-how to create a stylish ponytail.

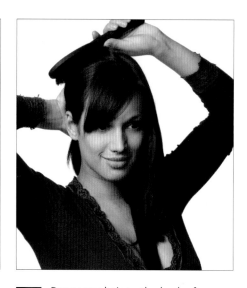

1 Brush dry hair to be smooth and tangle-free.

2 Draw your hair to the back of your head with a hairbrush and grasp with one hand to hold in place.

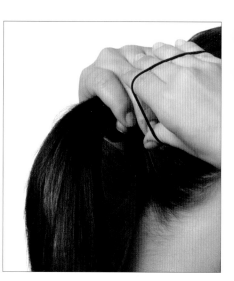

3 Secure the ponytail with a hairband (headband). A covered hairband rather than an elastic band is best if you have one as it doesn't snag and pull out hair as easily.

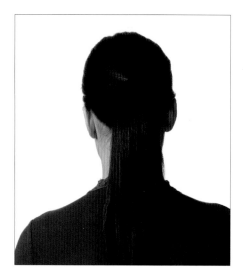

4 Here the ponytail is centrally placed with the base at the mid-point at the back of the head.

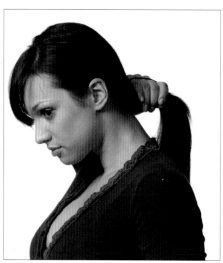

5 Alternatively, for a low tail, tip your head forward and draw the hair to the back of your head. This will position the base of the tail closer to the nape of your neck.

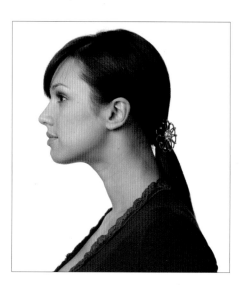

6 This is how the perfect low ponytail should look. Dress up the ponytail by using a decorative hairband (headband), if you like.

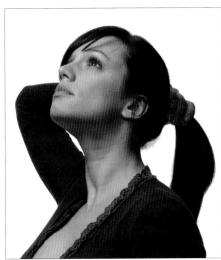

7 For a high ponytail, tip your head back and draw the hair to the back of your head. This places the base of the tail higher up the back of the head.

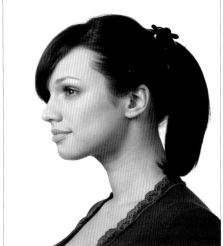

8 This is how the perfect high ponytail should look.

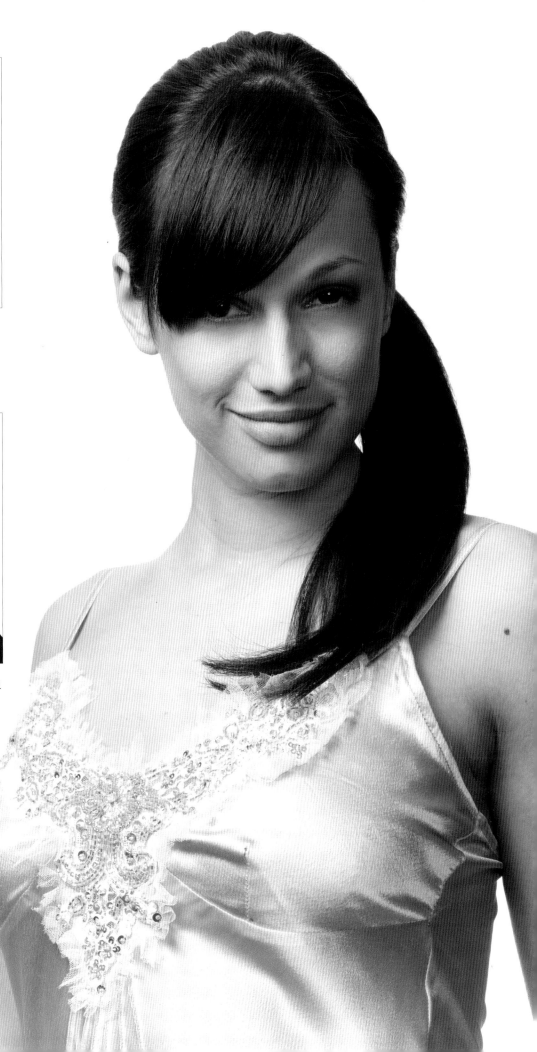

Stylist's note

Take a look at your profile and figure out where best to position a ponytail to complement your head shape.

Creating a perfect plaited ponytail

The technique is simple, but getting a plait to look even and neat is quite an art. Once mastered, you can apply the method in any number of styles. Here is a straightforward plaited ponytail to get you started.

You will need
- Hairbrush
- Covered hairbands (headbands)
- Light-hold hairspray
- Shine spray
- Accessories (optional)

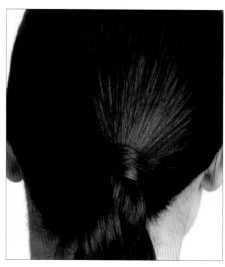

1 Brush dry hair to be tangle-free, then draw your hair into a ponytail at the back of the head, using a covered hairband (headband) to secure it.

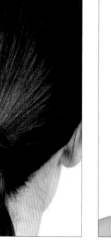

2 Wrap a small section of hair around the hairband at the base of the ponytail for a cleaner finish.

3 Spritz your hair all over with a light-hold hairspray. Don't overdo it or it may make the hair hard to work with – simply spritz spray above the head and allow it to settle on the hair.

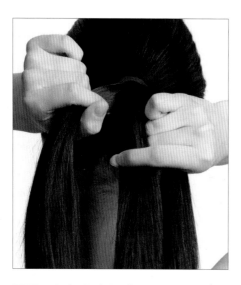

4 Divide the loose hair of the ponytail into three even sections.

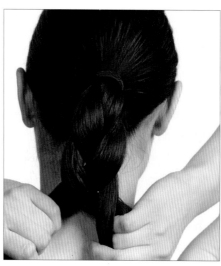

5 Weave the three sections together – taking left over centre, then right over centre and repeating.

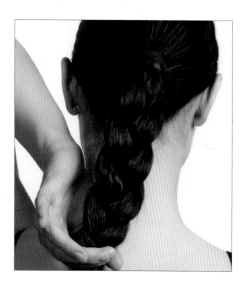

6 Continue to weave the hair into a plait (braid) until shortly before the ends of the sections.

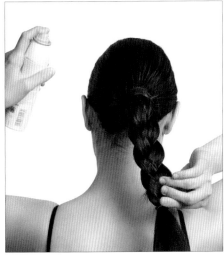

7 Secure the ends with a hairband and spray the plait with shine spray.

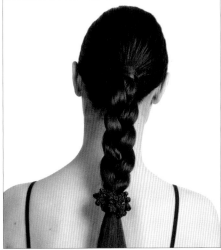

8 Add accessories to the end of the plait if you like, depending on the occasion.

Stylist's note

Using a light-hold spray before weaving the plait (braid) will calm flyaways and give a neater finish.

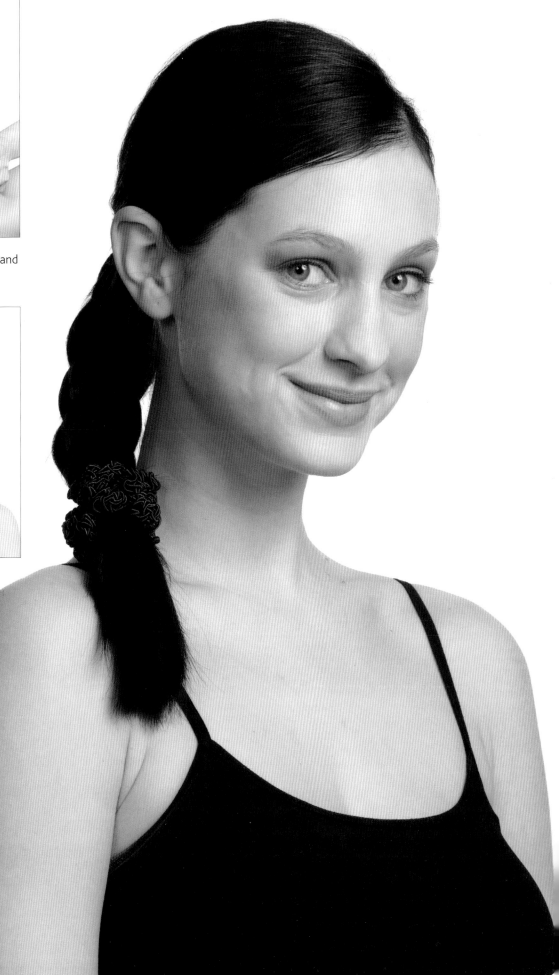

Creating a perfect ballerina bun

Neat and elegant, the ballerina bun is perfectly suited to a dancer who needs to create beautiful lines and keep hair off her face, and it creates a classic look at other times, too. Once in place, you can accessorize in any number of ways.

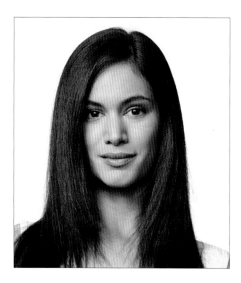

1 Brush dry hair to be completely tangle-free and smooth.

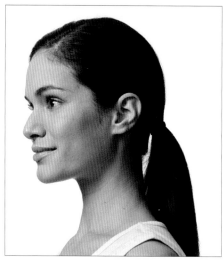

2 Draw your hair into a ponytail at the nape of your neck or slightly offset for an individual touch. Secure with a hairband (headband) and spray with hairspray for hold.

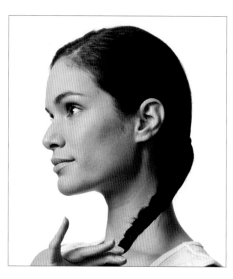

3 Take all the free ends of the tail and gently twist them together.

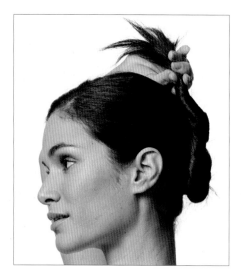

4 Continue twisting more tightly at the back of the head.

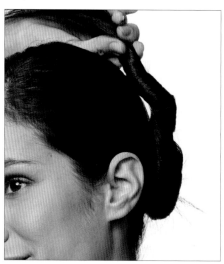

5 The tail will start to turn around itself as you continue twisting.

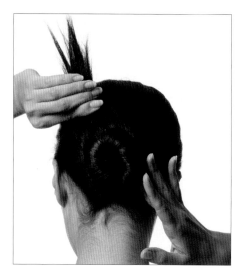

6 Wrap the twisted ends of the tail around the base of the ponytail and grip in place.

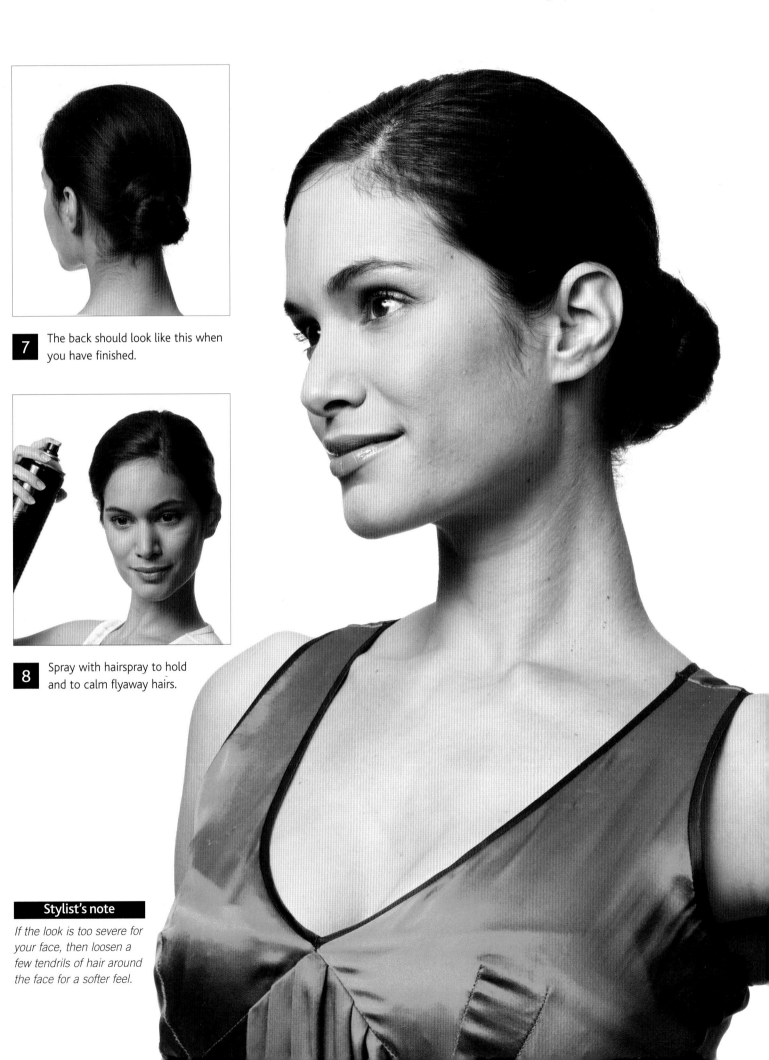

7 The back should look like this when you have finished.

8 Spray with hairspray to hold and to calm flyaway hairs.

Stylist's note

If the look is too severe for your face, then loosen a few tendrils of hair around the face for a softer feel.

Creating a perfect French roll

You will need
- Hairbrush
- Wide, open hair pins
- Hairspray
- Accessories (optional)

A chignon by any other name, this is a great up-do that can be dressed to be as chic and sophisticated as you like, or worn looser and casual for a more relaxed vibe. You can add accessories to suit any occasion.

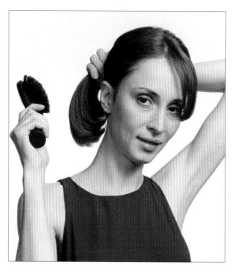

1 Brush dry hair to be smooth and tangle-free.

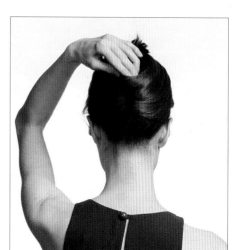

2 Draw your hair back into a ponytail with the base slightly to one side of your head at the back, and hold with your hand.

3 Without securing the ponytail with a hairband (headband), twist the hair being held so that it turns round and up to lie flat against the back of your head, forming the roll shape.

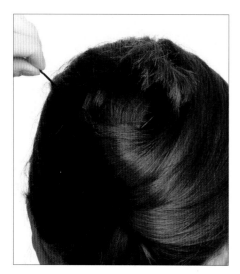

4 Pin the roll in place using open-ended pins, pushing the heads in as far as possible so they don't stick out.

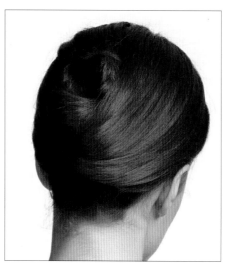

5 The roll should look like this from the back when you have finished pinning the hair.

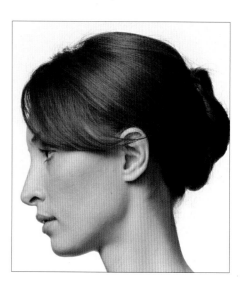

6 The hair should look like this from the side when you have finished pinning the hair.

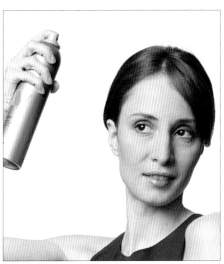

7 Spritz your hair with hairspray for hold and shine.

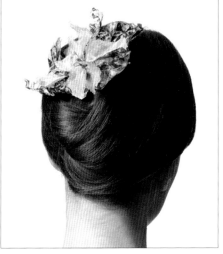

8 Add accessories if you like, depending on the occasion.

Stylist's note

Use open pins to secure the hair – as many as you like, provided they are pushed in firmly to conceal them as much as possible.

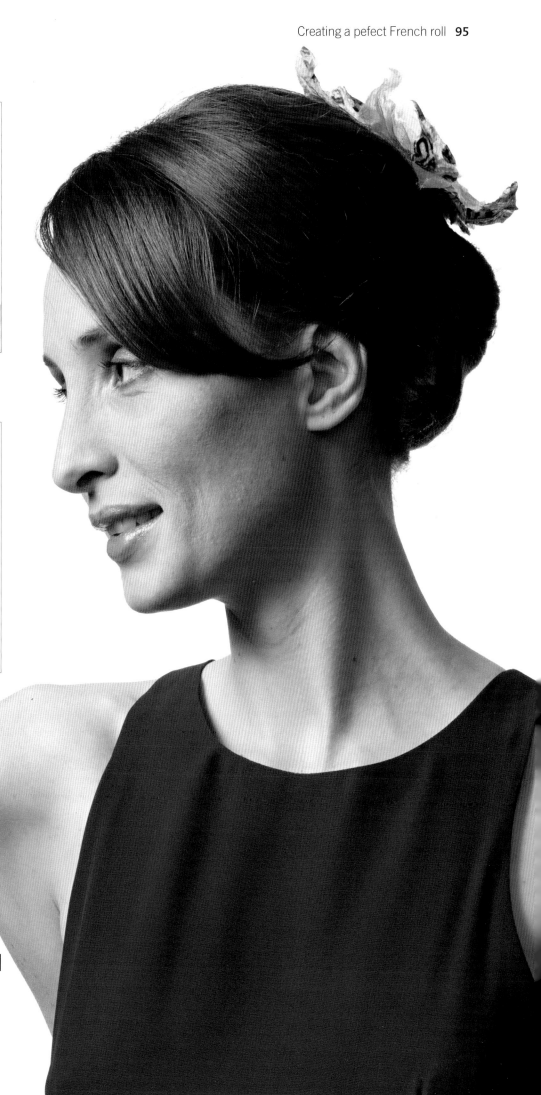

Creating a perfect woven bun

A simple ballerina bun can look more interesting if you work your hair into a plait first. It's perhaps easier to pin up too, especially when you are working with layered hair, which can be more tricky to style.

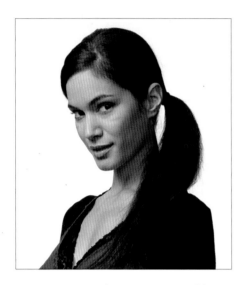

1 Draw your hair into a reasonably tight ponytail at the back of your head, slightly off centre, with an off-centre parting at the front. Secure in place with a covered hairband (headband).

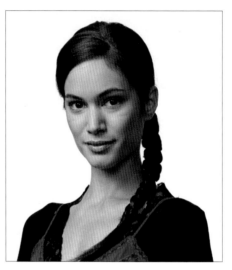

2 Weave the ends of the ponytail into a plait (braid) and secure the ends with a hairband.

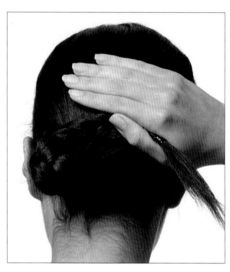

3 Wrap the plait around the base of the ponytail.

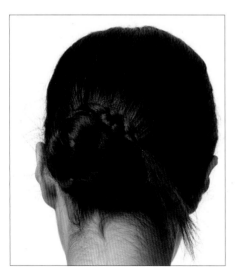

4 Grip the plait in place to form the bun shape.

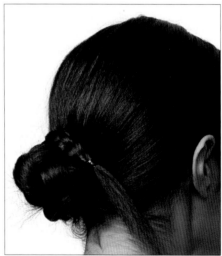

5 The smaller end of the plait should sit at the top of the bun as this will accentuate the detail of the weave better.

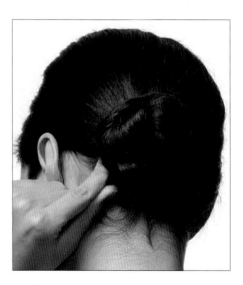

6 Tuck the free ends of the plait into the bun to hide them, and pin in place with hairgrips (bobby pins).

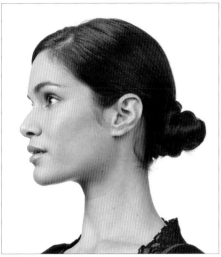

7 This is how the bun should look from the side when you have finished pinning it.

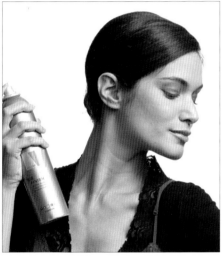

8 Spray with hairspray to hold and to calm flyaway hairs.

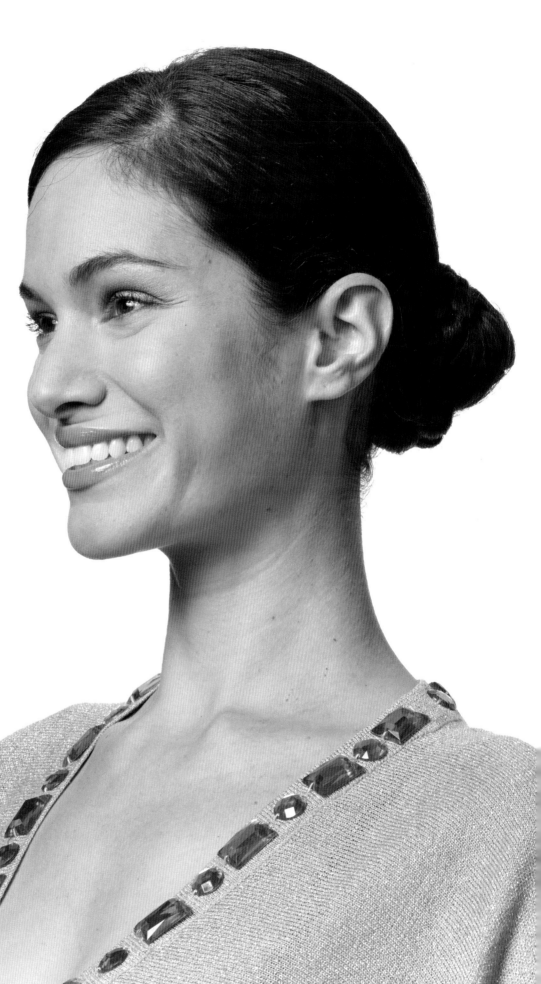

Stylist's note

Positioning a bun or ponytail to sit slightly to one side always adds an individual touch.

Creating a perfect French pleat

This is a gorgeous classic look that is particularly good for styling hair that is layered. Once you have mastered the technique, you can choose to pleat hair vertically, off-set or even horizontally for an individual touch.

You will need
- Hairbrush
- Covered hairband (headband)
- Hairspray
- Accessories (optional)

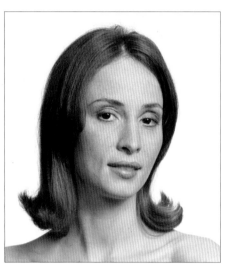

1 Brush dry hair to be tangle-free and completely smooth.

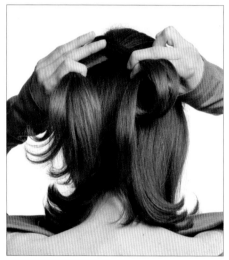

2 Starting at the top of the back of your head, take three even sections of hair from a central point and start to weave a plait (braid).

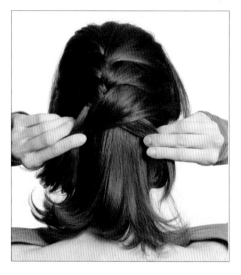

3 After one or two weaves, draw in small sections of loose hair from the sides as you continue the plait. You should incorporate all the hair from the sides as you go.

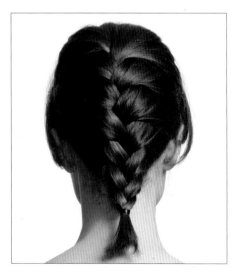

4 Secure the plait with a hairband (headband) when you reach the bottom of your hair.

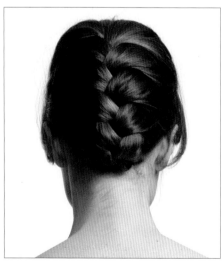

5 Tuck the free ends and any length of plait under the main body of the plait and pin to hold securely.

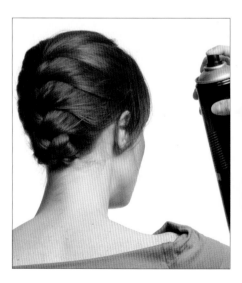

6 Spritz your hair with hairspray to hold and to keep the look neat.

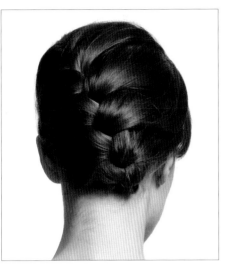

7 Alternatively, weave a plait from one side of the top area of your head to the opposite bottom side to form an offset French pleat (roll).

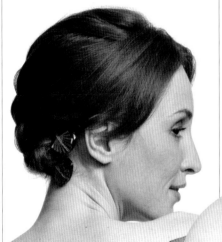

8 Add ornamental pins or other hair accessories for effect, if you like.

Stylist's note

The first time you try this style, position a mirror in front of you and one behind so you can see how the pleat (roll) is forming.

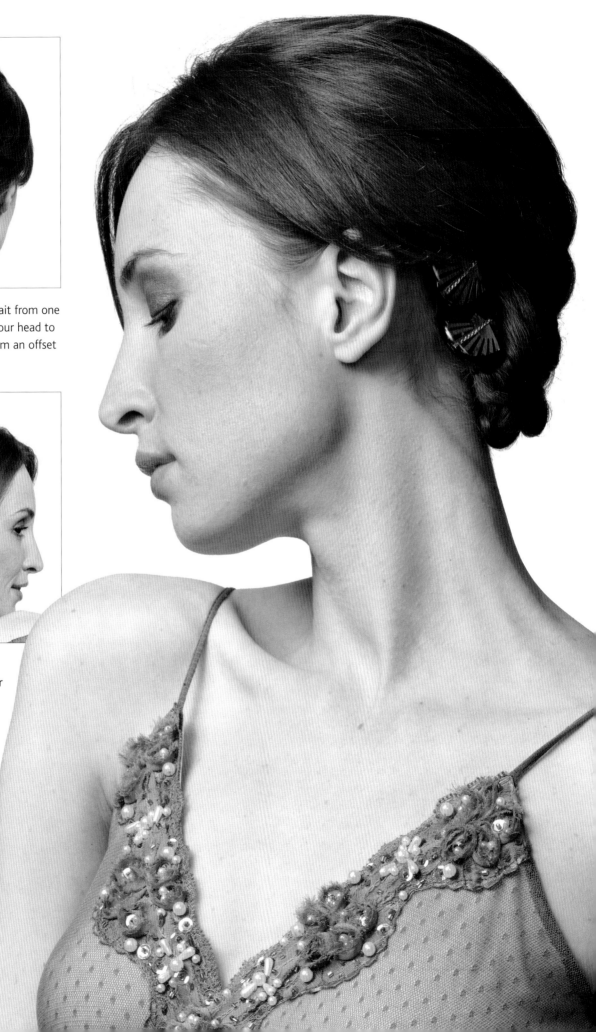

Creating a sweet asymmetric back-do

For a dressy style that offers a new and different take on a ponytail, this offset, drawn-back do is perfect. It leaves some hair to nestle around the neck for a softer line, yet is sleek-looking and sophisticated at the same time.

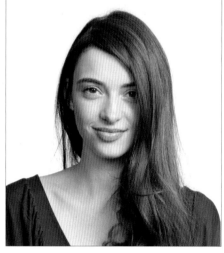

1 Brush clean, dry hair to be smooth and tangle-free.

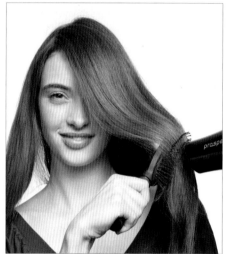

2 Using a paddle brush and a hairdryer work the hair to be as smooth as possible by brushing down the hair as you apply heat.

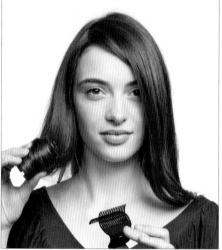

3 Place heated rollers in the hair but only wind through about three turns (depending on the length of hair) to stop in the mid-length area.

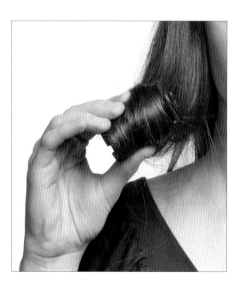

4 Use the rollers' own grips, pins or clasps to hold them in place and allow the rollers to cool completely.

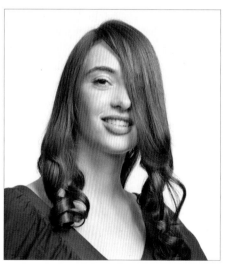

5 Remove all the clips and the rollers from your hair.

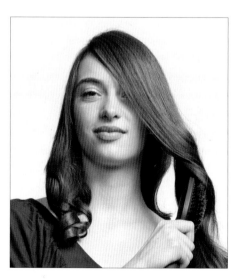

6 Lightly brush your hair to loosen but not lose the curl.

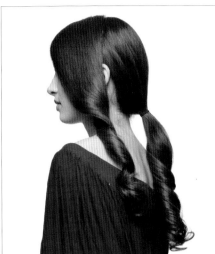

7 Part your hair down one side from centre front to the back of your ear. Secure the bigger section in a low ponytail leaving the other section free.

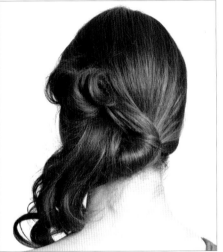

8 Take the loose section of hair and draw it back to go under then round over the base of the ponytail. Pin it in place so it disguises the band and so that all the free ends of hair tumble together.

Stylist's note

This look requires super-smooth hair, so it's important to work in extra smoothness using a hairbrush and a medium-heat setting on a hairdryer, even on dry hair.

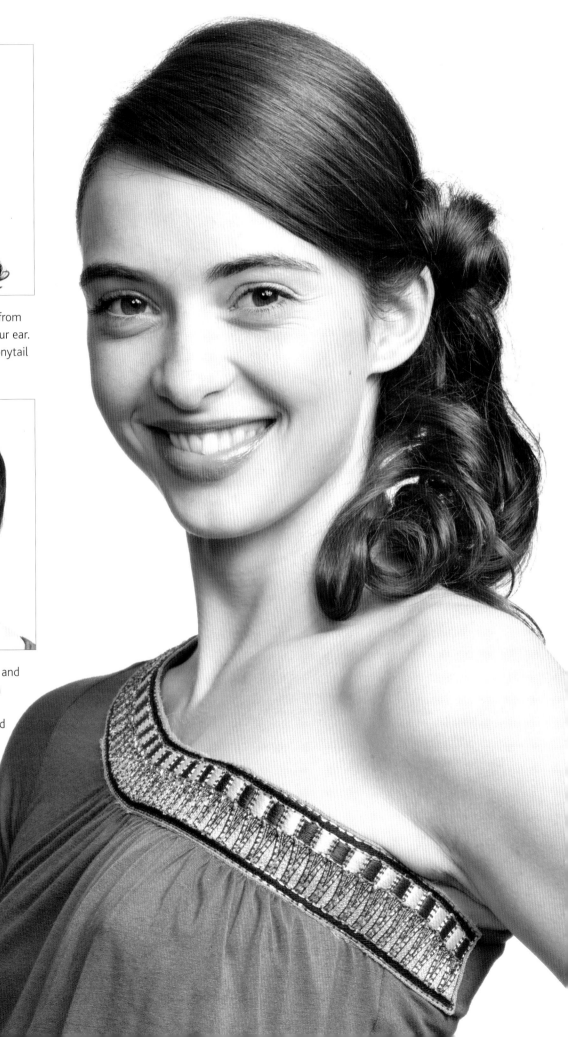

Creating a textured twist up-do on longer hair

You will need
- Hairdryer
- Sectioning clips
- Hairgrips (bobby pins)
- Open-ended pins
- Dressing-out brush
- Hairspray

It's fun to put long hair up into a style that suits both day and night. Rather than smoothing your hair into a really groomed up-do, work with the natural texture of the hair and don't be afraid of leaving ends free for a softer edge to finish.

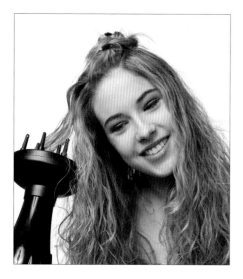

1 Diffuse-dry clean, long hair for added texture and volume. (See pages 32–3.)

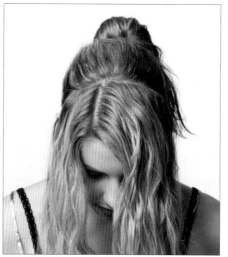

2 Section your hair from ear to ear across the top of your head using sectioning clips to form front and back sections, as shown here.

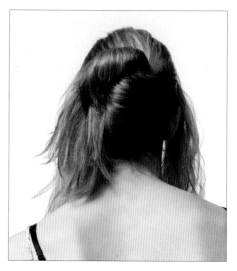

3 Grasp the hair from the back section and twist it up to lie against the back of your head, then turn the ends over to lie as shown. Grip in place with hairgrips (bobby pins).

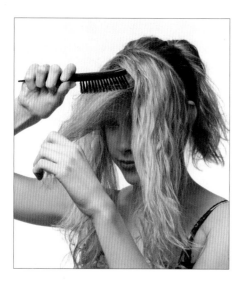

4 Taking the front section, backbrush the hair near the roots using a dressing-out brush.

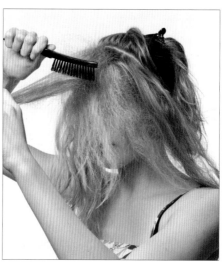

5 Continue to backbrush, taking hair from the front hairline and working backwards to the line where the front section finishes.

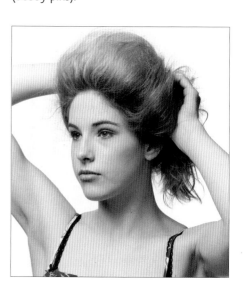

6 Lift and draw over the whole front section to the back of the head. You should now have a lot of height in the front section.

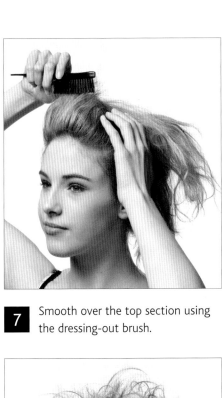

7 Smooth over the top section using the dressing-out brush.

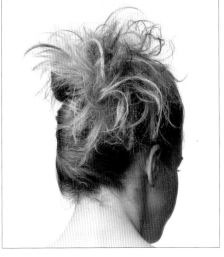

8 Pin this lifted and backbrushed front section at the back, placing it over the top of the twist created in Step 3. It should look like this. Spray with hairspray to hold.

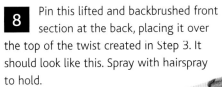

Stylist's note

You'll need to practise this a few times but once mastered, it's quick to do.

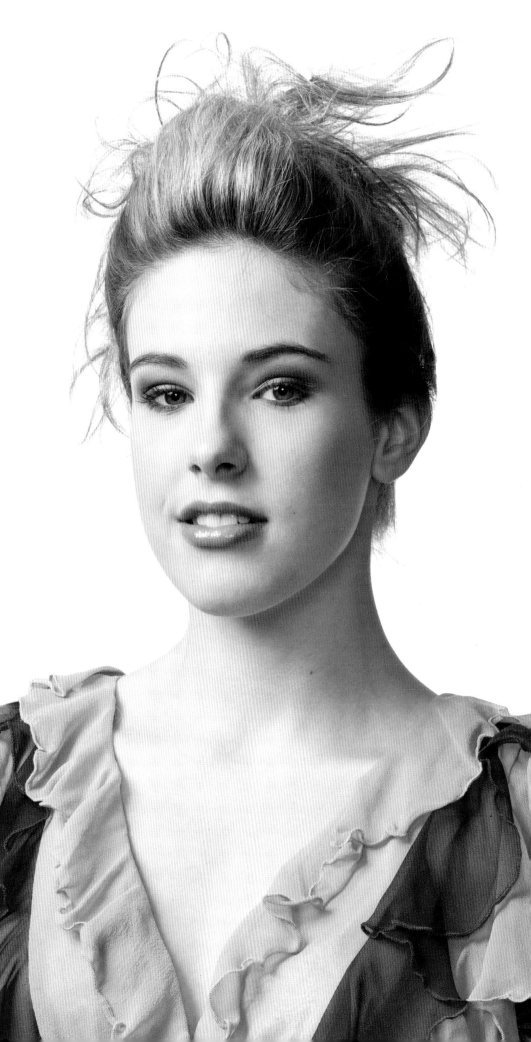

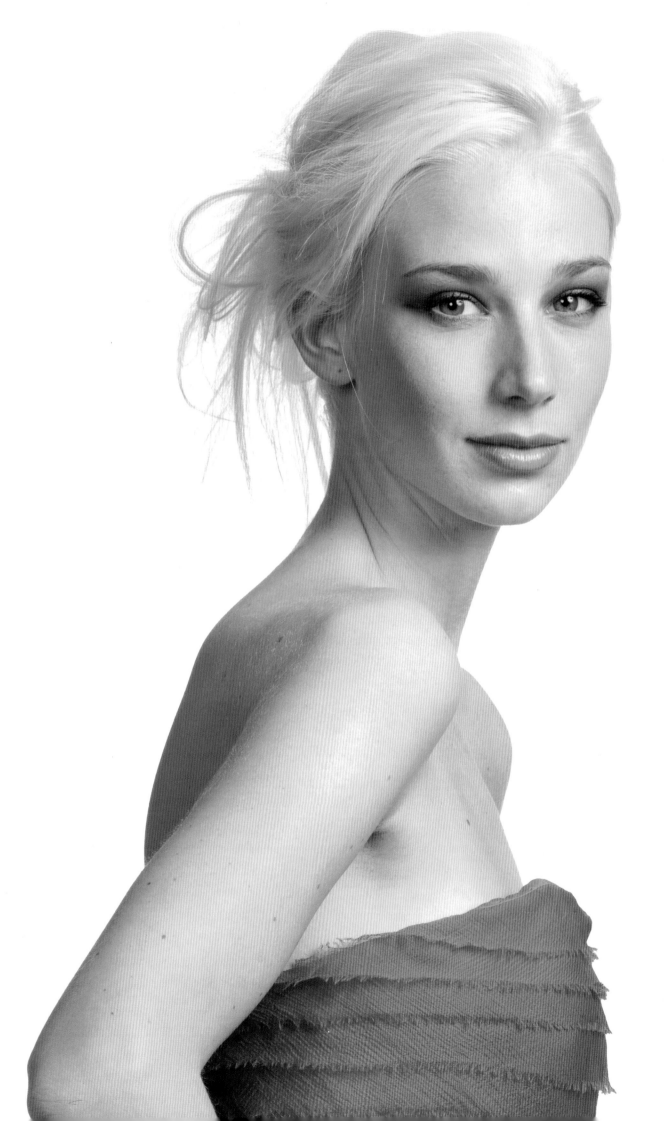

Special occasions

For those red-letter days when you really need a hairstyle with 'wow' factor, dress your hair in one of our special occasion dos. Whether you opt for elegance and classic chic or prefer to go for a sophisticated, contemporary style, the art of creating a fantastic look lies in being confident that your style suits you and will stay in place as long as you need it to. Take your time to practise the techniques so that when you come to the big day you will be calm and more than able to finish the hair superbly.

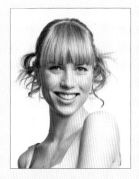 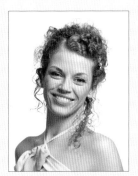 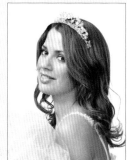

Creating a sleek, elegant finish on shorter hair

A shorter hair cut can be groomed to look just as special as an up-do on longer hair assuming you're prepared to channel effort into meticulous preparation and to select the right finishing products to show off your style.

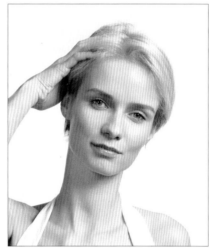

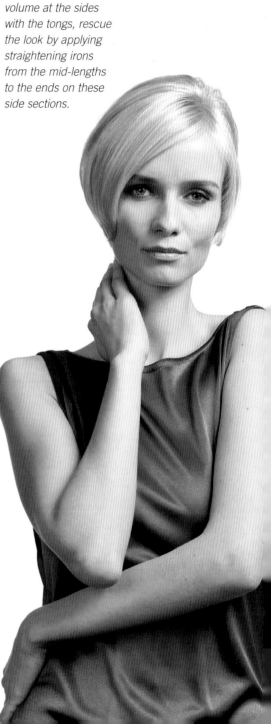

Stylist's note

If you find you have created too much volume at the sides with the tongs, rescue the look by applying straightening irons from the mid-lengths to the ends on these side sections.

1 Brush clean, dry hair to be smooth and tangle-free.

2 Put some styling lotion in the palm of one hand, rub your hands together and apply the lotion all over with your fingers, to protect your hair from heat and help to style it.

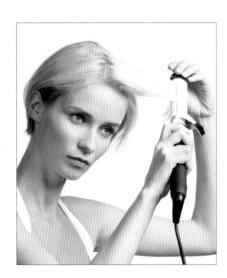

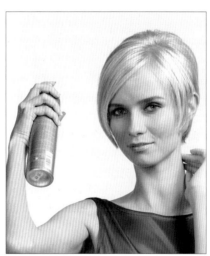

3 Taking sections of hair from the top of your head, place large-barrelled tongs at the ends of the hair and roll up to the roots. This will require one or two turns.

4 When all the hair has been tonged this way, brush through and smooth into shape. Spritz all over with hairspray for hold and shine spray to finish.

Creating a glamorous pin-up on shorter curly hair

You will need
- Hairgrips (bobby pins)
- Hairspray

If you are in need of a great evening look but time isn't on your side, or you don't have much in the way of styling equipment, then curly hair can quickly be pinned into a simple yet effective style that will make you a real belle of the ball.

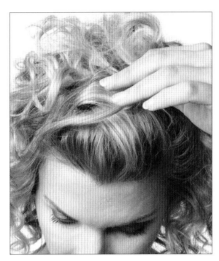

> **Stylist's note**
>
> *Grip each new section of hair that is drawn back so that it conceals the hairgrip (bobby pin) inserted to hold the previous piece of hair.*

1 Lift a small section of hair from one side at the front. Draw it back and over towards the opposite side and grip securely in place. Repeat with the other side.

2 Continue to lift and pin hair from one side to the other to build shape and draw hair off your face.

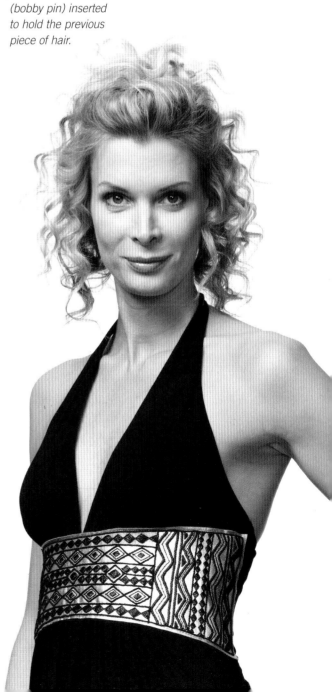

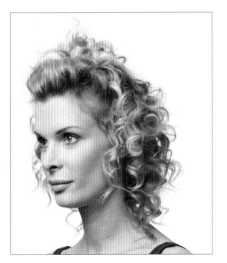

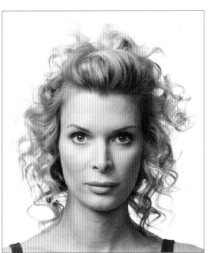

3 Don't clip too much back – you should leave the side area loose as the curls will soften and frame your face.

4 When you have finished clipping, your hair should be drawn off your forehead and show a little bit of height on top. Spritz with light-hold spray to finish the look.

Creating a quick, chic party look on shorter hair

For the times when you have to move quickly from office to party without the luxury of being able to get ready at home, this look is cool yet sophisticated and special enough to wear with any smart evening outfit.

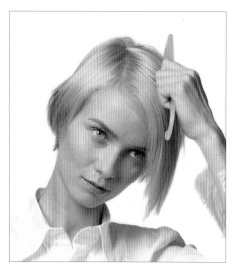

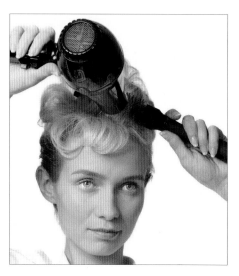

1 Comb dry hair to be tangle-free and to remove any products that may have been applied earlier in the day.

2 Comb through your hair again so it is smooth and spritz all over with styling lotion.

3 Section out the top area of hair. Wrap small sections of hair, one at a time, round a small-barrelled round brush and blast with heat from a hairdryer.

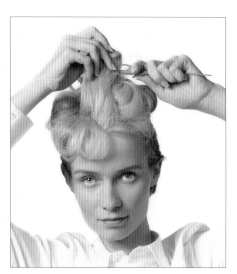

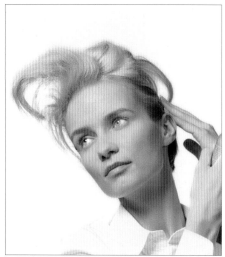

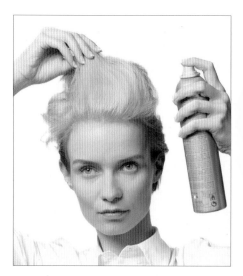

4 When cool, back-comb the hair in the top section at the roots to create height and texture.

5 Smooth back the hair at the sides and spritz with strong-hold hairspray to keep in place.

6 Mould the top section to form a quiff shape and spray to hold, particularly at the roots.

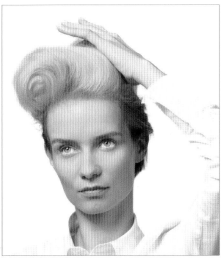

7 Use the palm of your hand to smooth over the hair and accentuate this quiff shape.

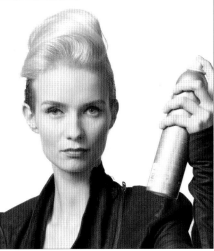

8 Spritz your hair again all over with hairspray for hold, and shine spray to finish.

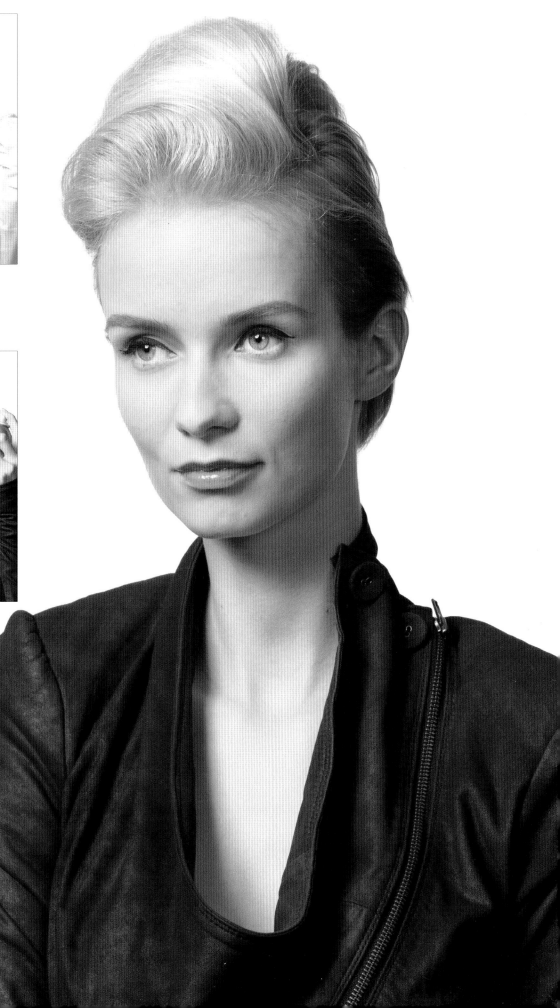

Creating a quick party look on mid-length hair

It's challenging moving straight from work to a special occasion without all your styling tools to hand. Here's a quick look that can be achieved with a travel-sized hairdryer and a round brush and have you looking great in no time.

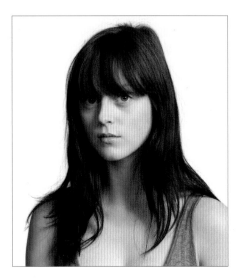

1 Brush dry hair to be completely tangle-free and smooth.

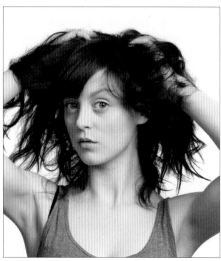

2 Rub styling lotion into the root area with your fingers to add lift and movement to the hair.

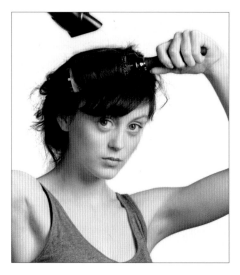

3 Wrap sections of hair around a round brush to create volume and apply heat from a hairdryer.

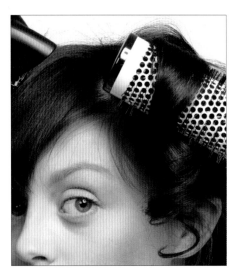

4 A ceramic round brush works particularly well here.

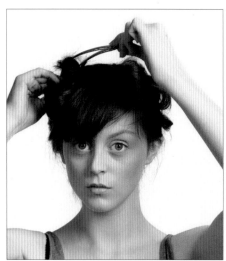

5 Using sectioning clips, secure each wrap in place while the hair cools.

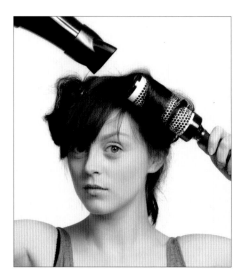

6 Work around the head, curling and pinning sections of hair but leaving a fringe (bangs) area out, if you have one. Leave for a few minutes to set.

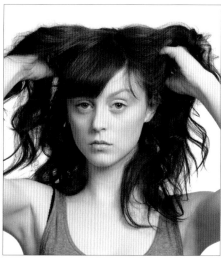

7 Remove the pins, then shake your hair loose and run your fingers through it.

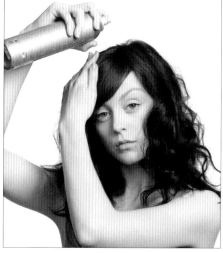

8 Spritz the smoother fringe area with shine spray.

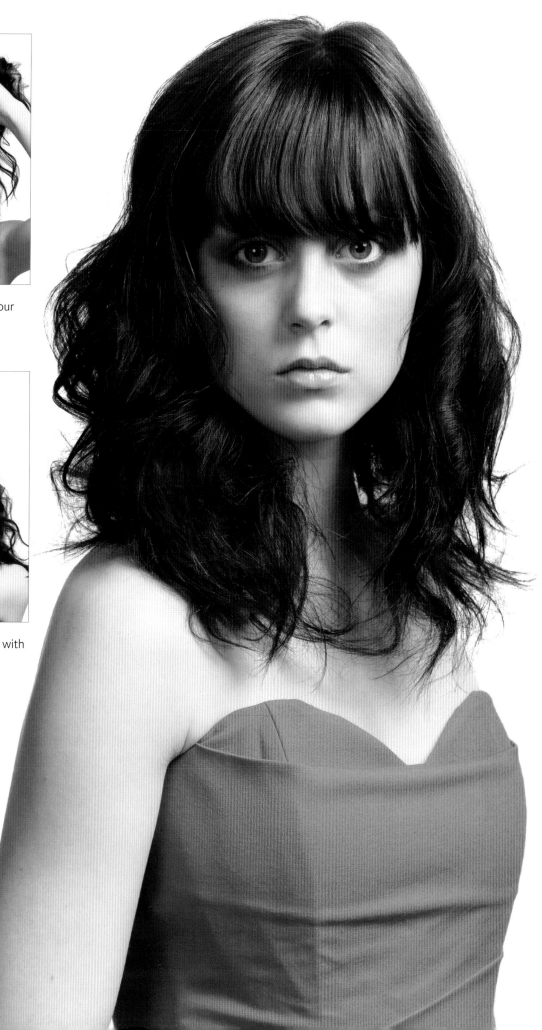

Creating a quick party look on curly hair

This look is very fast to put in place and once you know how to do it, you can make it your own by adding individual details such as ornaments. The technique can also be used on straight hair, which you can tong or crimp first for texture.

You will need
- Styling crème
- Smoothing crème
- Hairgrips (bobby pins)
- Open-ended pins
- Light-hold hairspray

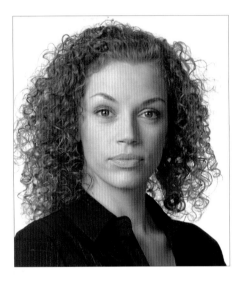

1 Start with clean hair that is dry. If you have straighter hair, curl or crimp it for added texture and volume.

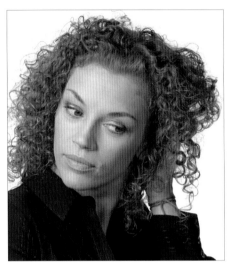

2 Apply a smoothing crème with your fingers to define curls and prevent your hair from frizzing.

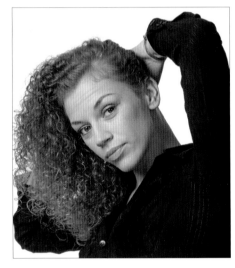

3 Push all your hair to one side of your head and hold in place with the flat of one hand. Hair at the front should go back and to the side, off your forehead, as shown.

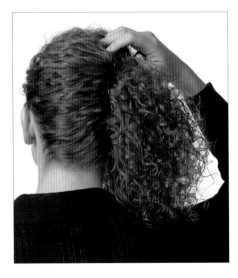

4 With the other hand, secure the hair at the back of the head using hairgrips (bobby pins) criss-crossed in a line down the back of the head.

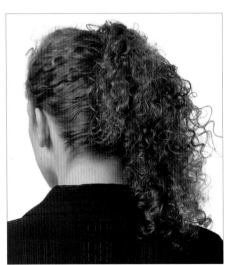

5 Arrange the hair at the back to fall so it covers these hairgrips. You can do this by twisting the top section of hair and pinning it again with open-ended pins.

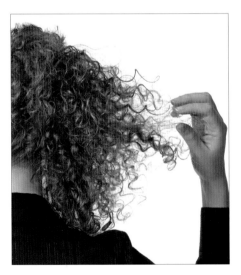

6 Using your fingers, loosen the free ends to encourage volume and apply more smoothing crème to define the curl, if necessary.

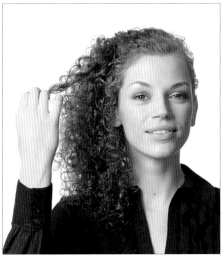

7 At the front, pull some tendrils of hair free around your face to soften the look.

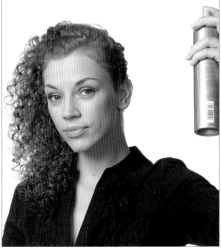

8 Spritz your hair all over with a light-hold hairspray to finish.

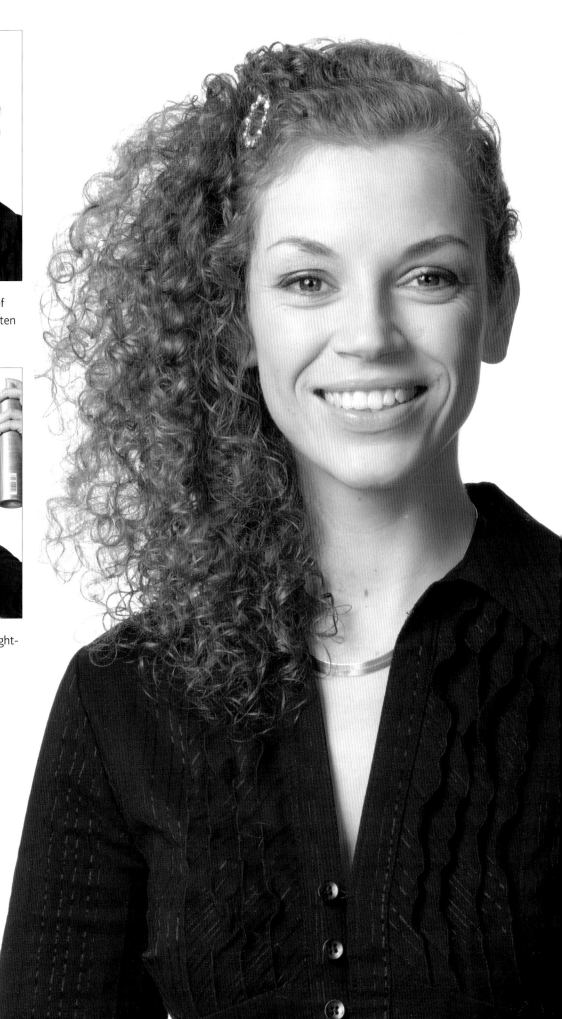

Stylist's note

By criss-crossing hairgrips (bobby pins) you will make the hold more secure.

Creating a perfect wave set

Show off a glorious mane of superbly conditioned hair with a stylish set using heated rollers. It's a look that is sexy and alluring if done well. Enhance with finishing products that bring out the natural shine of your hair.

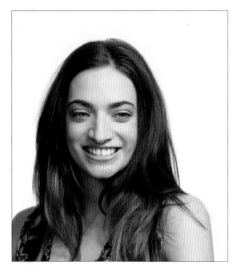

1 Plug in the heated rollers. Brush clean, dry hair with a hairbush to be completely tangle-free, then spritz all over with setting spray, which will help the waves stay in your hair.

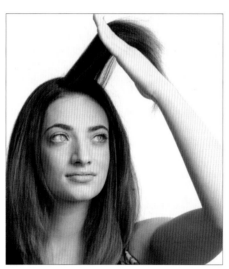

2 Starting at the middle top front of your head, take a section of hair in your hand.

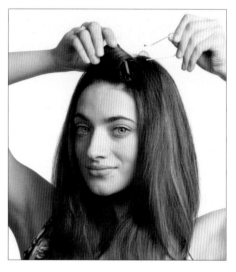

3 Wrap this hair around a heated roller and grip in place.

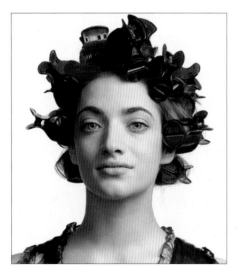

4 Continue to work through your hair from the front to the back and through the sides until all your hair is wound in rollers and gripped in place.

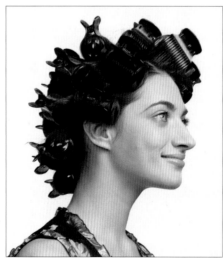

5 Your hair should look like this when you have finished.

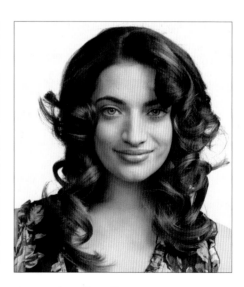

6 When the rollers are cool, remove the hairgrips (bobby pins) and take out the rollers.

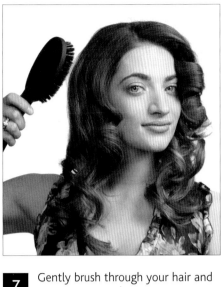

7 Gently brush through your hair and style how you like.

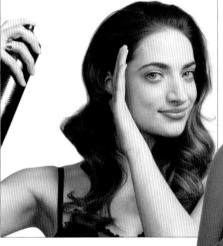

8 Apply a touch of serum to bring out the curl and spritz all over with shine spray and a light-hold hairspray.

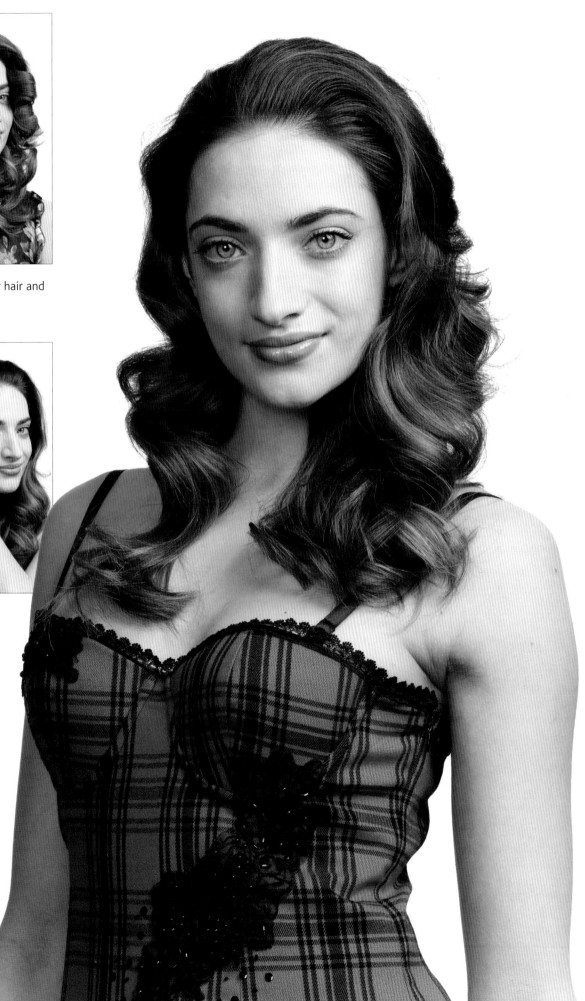

Stylist's note

Work from the top of your head down when putting in the heated rollers – there's no need to section hair first.

Creating sumptuous curls on straight hair

Transform straight hair into a mass of curls that balance a sophisticated evening dress and look soft and pretty yet grown up and alluring, too. Then simply pin up sections of hair to create a shape and you're fit to go.

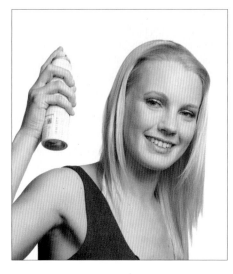

1 Comb dry hair to be smooth and spritz with heat-protective spray.

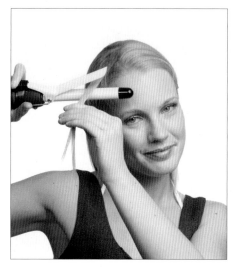

2 Starting at the top front of your head, and working small sections at a time, place curling tongs about one third of the way down the hair. Clamp the tongs shut.

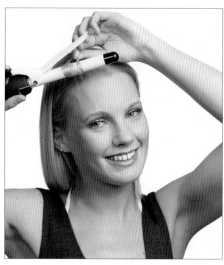

3 Wrap the hair round the barrel of the curling tongs down to the ends of the hair.

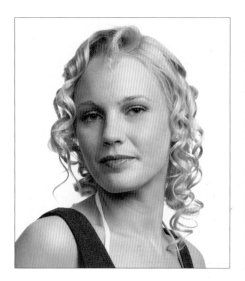

4 Work around the head in the same way so that hair is tonged all over.

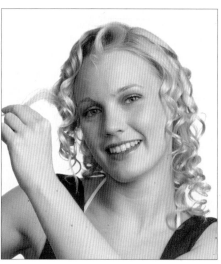

5 Loosen the curls using your fingers, then tease the hair.

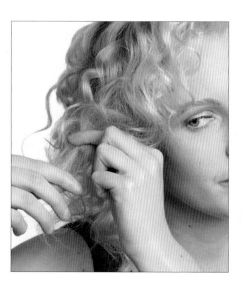

6 Work around your head loosening the curls with your fingers to create a beautiful soft finish.

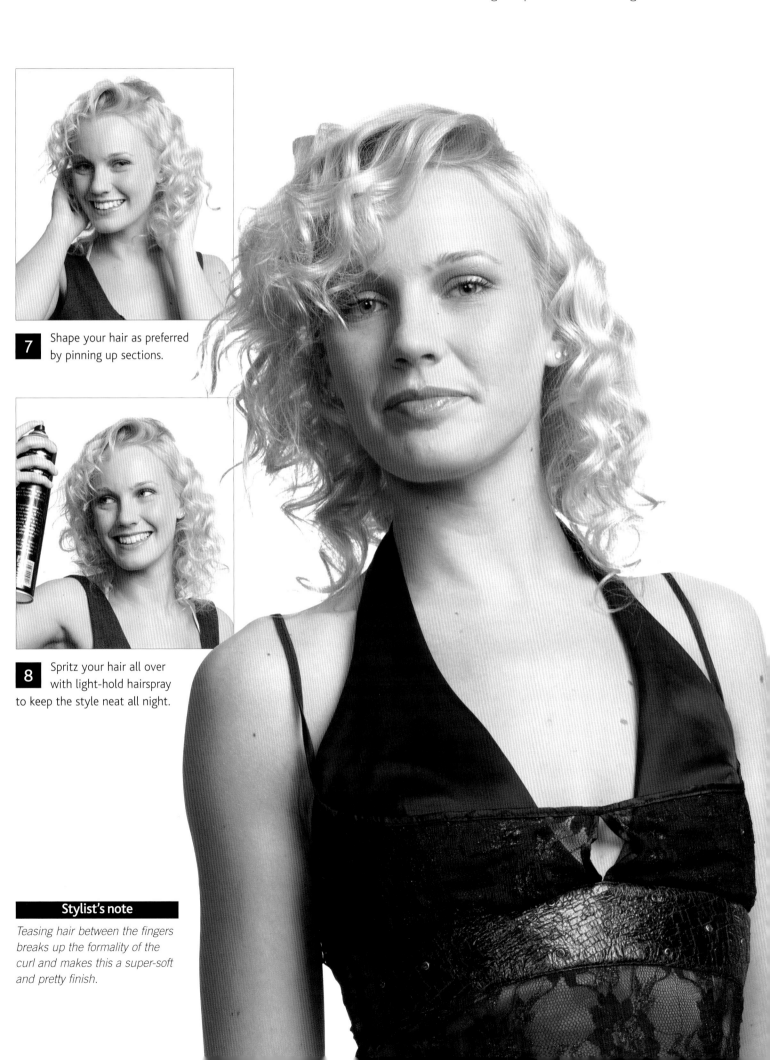

7 Shape your hair as preferred by pinning up sections.

8 Spritz your hair all over with light-hold hairspray to keep the style neat all night.

Teasing hair between the fingers breaks up the formality of the curl and makes this a super-soft and pretty finish.

Creating sophisticated ponytails for special events

There are plenty of ways to add interest to a ponytail and keep it fresh on any length hair without the need for ribbons and accessories. Here are a few ideas on how to create a really chic finish that looks good from every angle.

You will need
- Hairbrush
- Covered hairband (headband)
- Hairgrips (bobby pins)
- Hairspray
- Shine spray

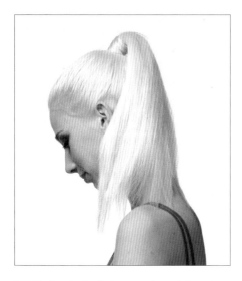

1 Brush dry hair smooth and draw it into a high ponytail at the back of your head. Secure with a covered hairband (headband), then wrap a piece of hair round the hairband to conceal it.

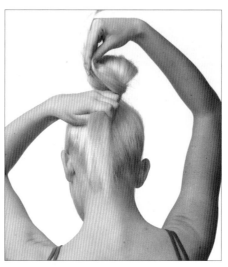

2 Lift most of the ponytail up and under to form a loop held against the base of the ponytail with your hand. Use the remaining hair to wrap around both the loop and all of the hairband.

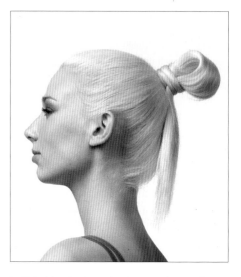

3 Pin the loop in place underneath so it is secure and the pins don't show.

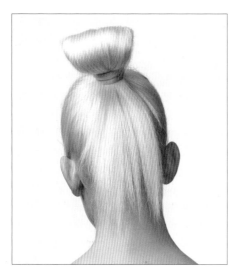

4 The ponytail should look like this when you have finished.

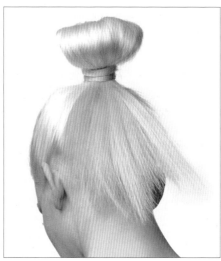

5 The free ends can be backbrushed to make a fantail and spritzed with hairspray to hold, if you like.

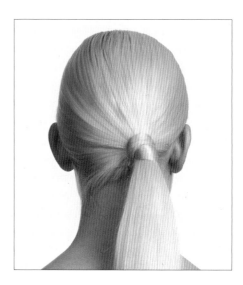

6 Alternatively, make a ponytail low at the base of your neck and positioned slightly off-centre.

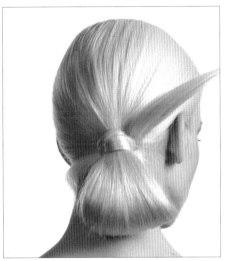

7 Roll the tail back under itself and grip in place, leaving one piece of the ponytail free to then wrap round the base and conceal the join.

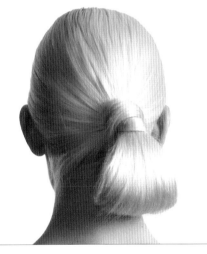

8 The end can be tucked into the base for a neater finish and pinned in place so it is secure. Spritz with shine spray to finish.

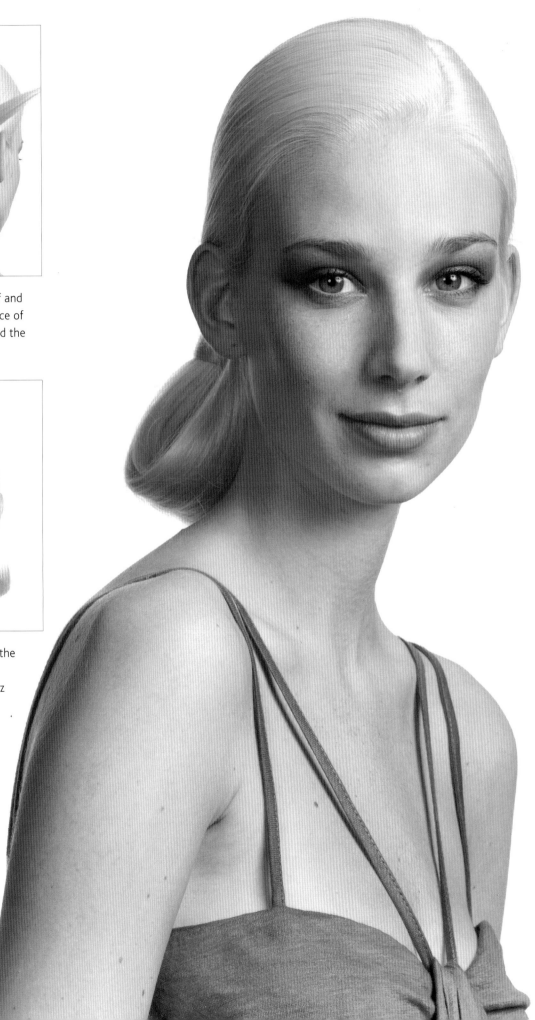

Creating a slick offset ballerina bun

For an individual look, put hair up into a classic bun but place it to one side and nearer the front than the back. Accessorize with an ornament or flower and you have a more contemporary take on a traditional style.

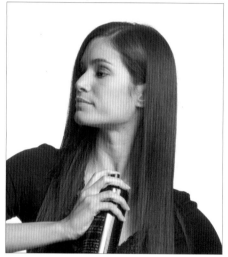

1 Brush dry hair to be completely smooth and tangle-free.

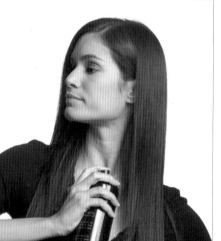

2 Apply hairspray throughout for added volume and hold.

3 Draw your hair into a reasonably tight ponytail with the base of the tail placed to one side of the front of the head, and secure in place with a covered hairband (headband).

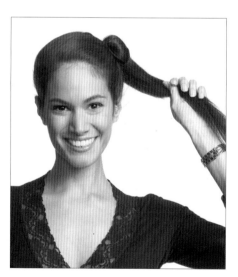

4 Twist the free ends of the ponytail until they wrap back around the base of the ponytail.

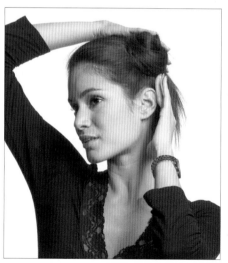

5 Grip the twisted bun into place with hairgrips (bobby pins) so it is secure.

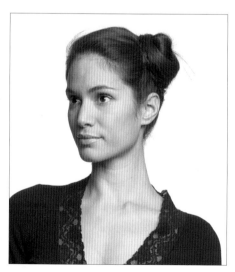

6 The bun should now look like this, with the end of the ponytail tucked in neatly.

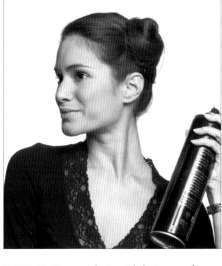

7 Spritz your hair with hairspray for hold and then shine spray to finish.

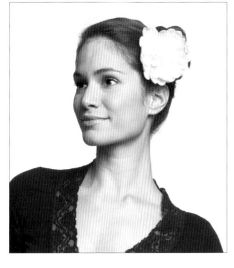

8 Add an accessory secured at the base of the bun for effect.

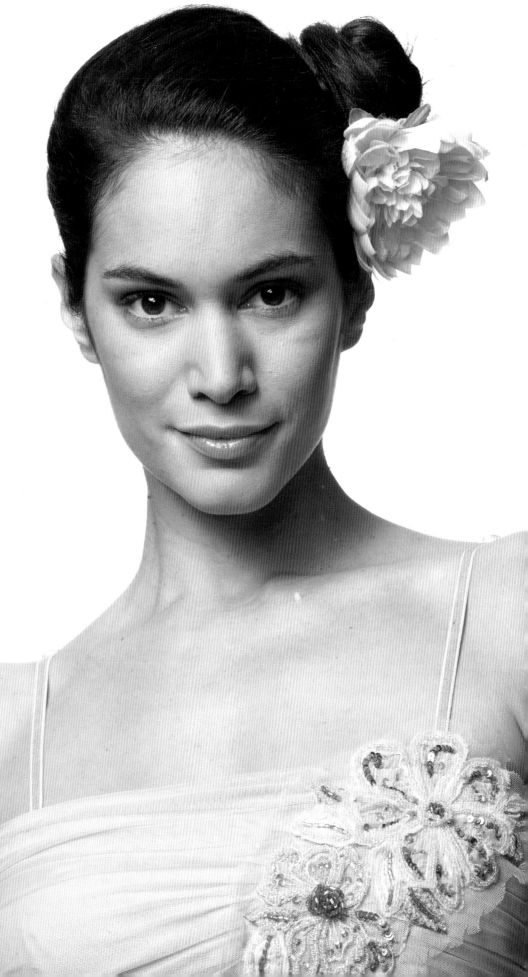

Stylist's note

This style relies on hair being long enough to sweep cleanly round from one side of the head to the other.

Creating a perfect classic chignon

So chic, sophisticated and timeless, a chignon is the perfect up-do for anyone wanting to exude a classic sense of style. You can wear it sleek and groomed or looser and accessorized for a more contemporary feel.

You will need
- Hairbrush
- Comb
- Hairspray
- Hairgrips (bobby pins)
- Open-ended pins
- Fine-waved pins

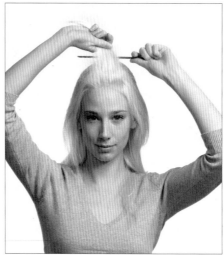

1 Brush dry hair to be completely tangle-free and smooth.

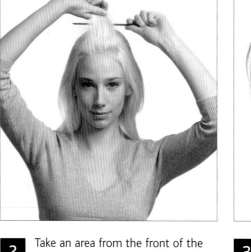

2 Take an area from the front of the top of your head to the top back and backbrush the roots with a comb to the mid-lengths of the hair.

3 Spritz all the hair that is back-brushed with hairspray to maintain the volume you have created. Draw back this top section and smooth the very top layer with the dressing-out brush.

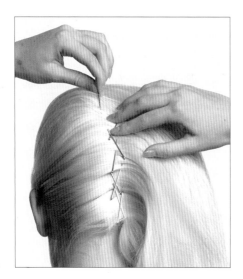

4 Sweep all the hair at the back horizontally to one side and grip in place with hairgrips (bobby pins) placed in a criss-cross pattern, as shown.

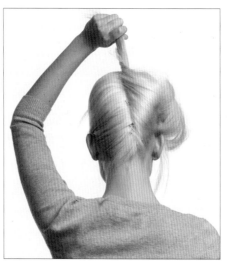

5 Take hold of the loose hair at the back from a point behind the ear. Twist it up to lie against the head. Use open-ended pins to secure along the edge.

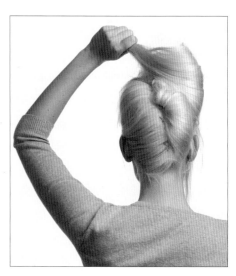

6 Take hold of the remaining loose hair from the front side. Twist it loosely and draw it across the back to blend in with the top of the previously pinned twist.

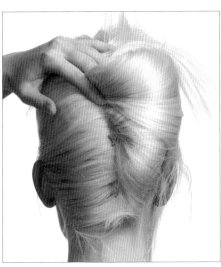

7 Use fine-waved pins to fix this third top section of hair securely in place (fine-waved pins are more easily concealed than standard pins).

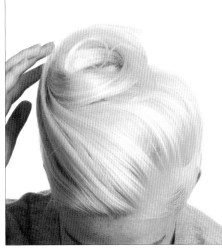

8 Tuck in any free ends so they curl inside the top of the chignon roll (use the tail of a comb to ensure all loose ends are tucked out of sight). Spray with hairspray to hold in place.

Stylist's note

You could use a dressing-out brush rather than a comb to create a cloud of angel hair, which adds volume to the chignon shape.

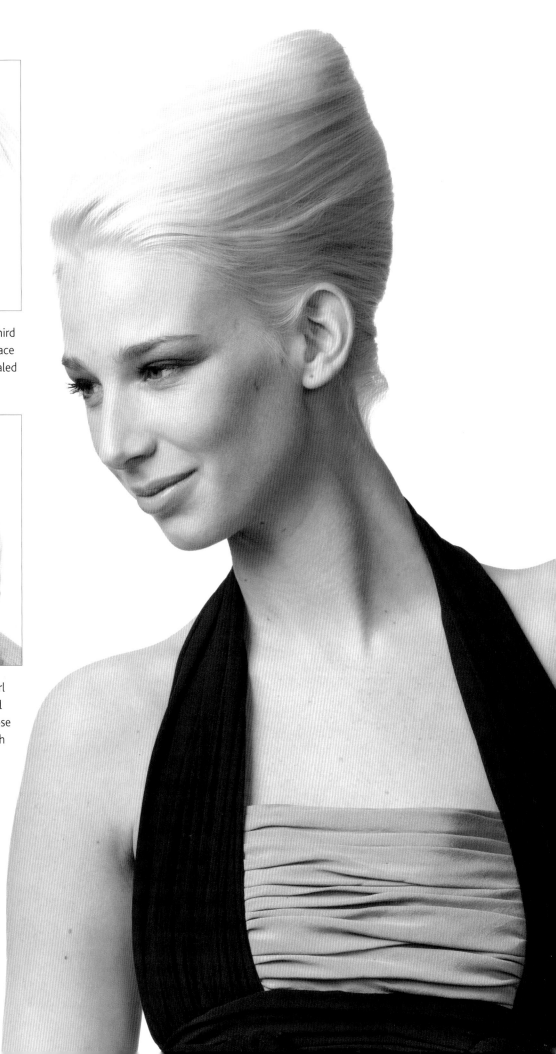

Creating a pin-up on mid-length hair

Pin hair up but leave a strong fringe in place to contrast with the texture at the back and to keep the look more relaxed and softer on the face. You can make the texture at the back as understated or exuberant as you like.

You will need
- Sectioning clips
- Hairbands (headbands)
- Curling tongs
- Hairgrips (bobby pins)
- Comb
- Hairspray

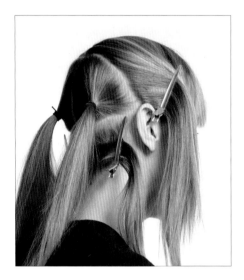

1 Section your hair from ear to ear across the top of the head with sectioning clips. Then section the hair from ear to ear across the back of the head. Centrally part each of the three sections.

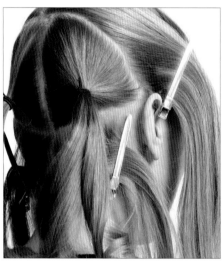

2 Secure the middle two back sections as ponytails with hairbands (headbands). Wrap hair round curling tongs to separate each ponytail into three spiral sections.

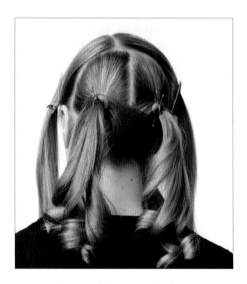

3 Lift one of the lower back sections to cross over to the opposite ponytail, wrap it around the base of the ponytail, then grip in place. Repeat on the other side. The back should now look like this.

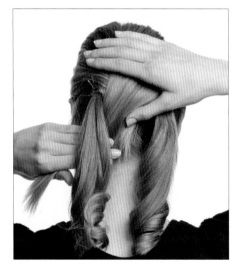

4 Bring each of the upper side sections in turn down to cross at the back of the head then to tuck under the ponytail on the opposite side.

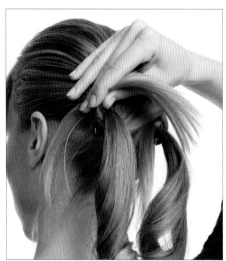

5 Bring the side sections back up to wrap around the base of the ponytail and tuck or grip the loose ends into the base of the ponytail, under the hairband.

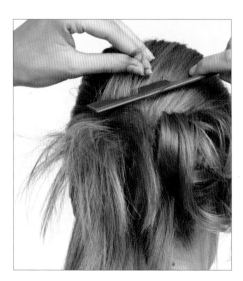

6 Back-comb each ponytail to add volume and texture.

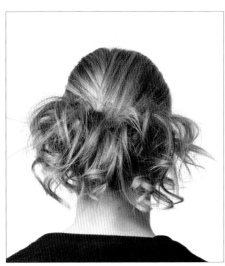

7 Fan out the ponytails slightly so the hair covers the gap in the middle at the back of your head.

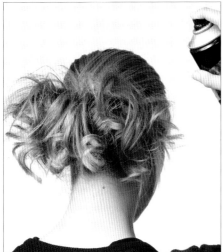

8 Spritz all of your hair with hairspray to hold.

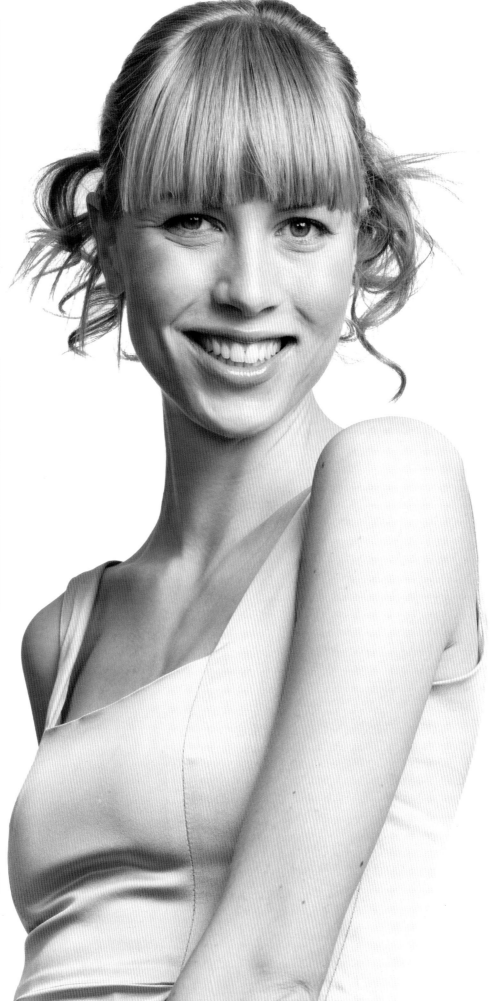

Stylist's note

Use black, dark brown or blonde hairgrips (bobby pins) according to your hair colour so they are easier to hide.

Creating a twist back-do on mid-length hair

When it seems as though all the special up-dos are best worked on longer hair, here's a great little up-do that works brilliantly with mid-length hair and allows you to leave your fringe free, if you have one.

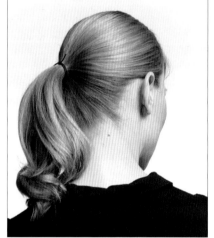

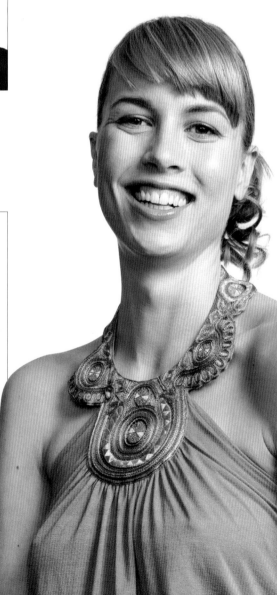

Stylist's note

When putting hair up it's best if it's 'day old hair', meaning that it has not been washed for 24 hours. This helps hairgrips (bobby pins) and pins to hold the style.

1 Brush clean, dry hair with a hairbrush to be completely tangle-free and smooth, then draw it into a reasonably tight ponytail at the back of the head in the middle.

2 Secure the ponytail with a hairband (headband).

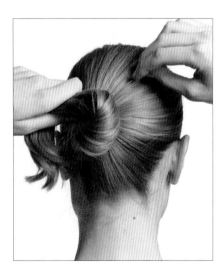

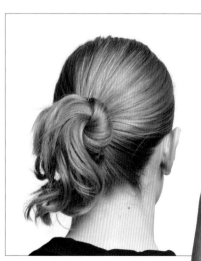

3 Grasp the free ends of the ponytail and twist to wrap it up round the base.

4 Grip the ponytail at the top and side and don't worry about loose ends and flyaways; it's part of the look.

Creating a twist up-do on longer hair

You will need
- Hairbrush
- Open-ended pins
- Hairspray

To contrast with a formal dress, it can be charming to create an up-do that balances an ultra-groomed outfit with a relaxed, softer finish for your hair. This twist up-do is really easy and works well on layered or fine and flyaway hair.

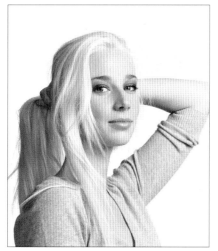

1 Brush clean, dry hair with a hairbrush to be tangle-free but not super-smooth, then loosely draw it back off the face leaving some hair hanging free at the front.

2 Loosely twist the hair at the back and turn it up so that it lies against the back of the head.

Stylist's note

Once pinned into place, you can continue to pull free tendrils of hair loose until you have the face-framing softness you prefer.

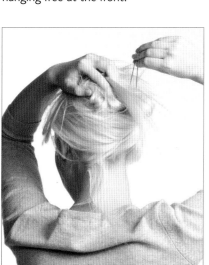

3 Pin the twisted hair into place using open-ended pins.

4 Work some ends into the pinned hair, but leave some hair free for a softer effect. Spritz liberally with hairspray to hold.

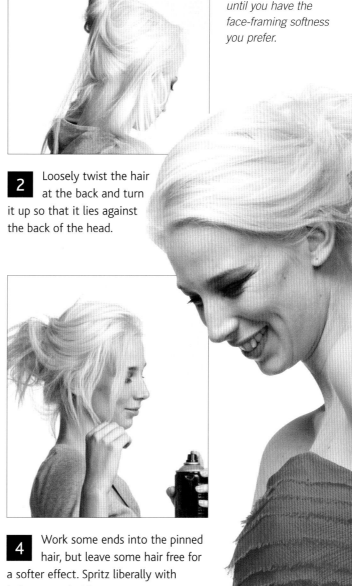

Creating a mussed-up back-do on mid-length hair

Bring out the colours in your hair with a back-do that is fabulously mussed-up and casual from behind yet groomed and styled at the front. It's individual and smart enough for any occasion without looking as though you have tried too hard.

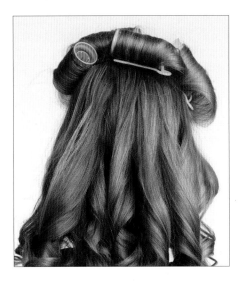

1 Plug in the heated rollers. Spritz dry hair with styling spray. Tong hair through the back using a spiral wind. Wrap the hair at the top of the head in four heated rollers (no more).

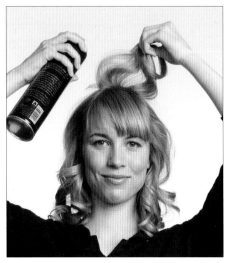

2 Remove the rollers when they are cool. Spritz the top section with hairspray at the roots to create lift (tip your head forwards for added volume).

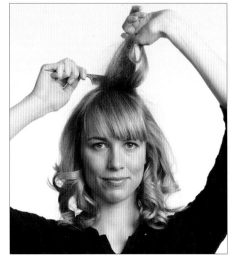

3 Take the top section of hair that was in rollers and gently backcomb the roots to add height. Grip it loosely out of the way at the top of the head.

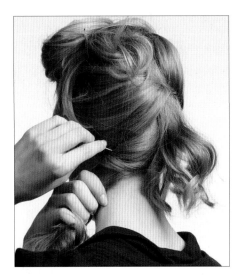

4 Lift the upper half of the back section, take this hair to one side and grip to hold. Lift the lower half of the back section and grip over to the other side.

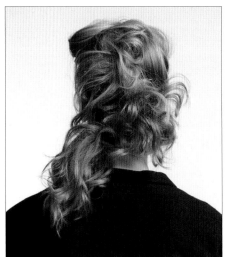

5 Your hair should now look like this, with just one piece of hair loose on one side. Spritz with hairspray to hold.

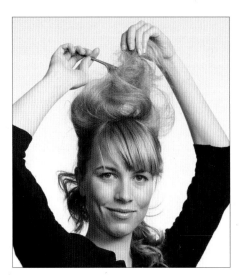

6 Return to the top section and backcomb the ends to create texture, then grip at the back, taking care to conceal hairgrips (bobby pins) as much as possible.

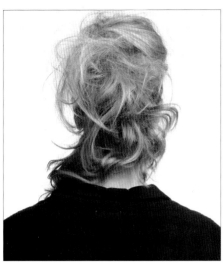

7 You can continue to backcomb and create as much texture as you like, working with the free ends but taking care not to dislodge grips.

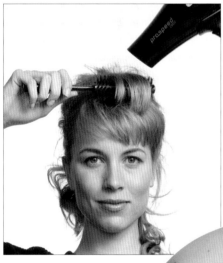

8 Blow-dry the fringe (bangs) area round a barrel brush for smoothness and to contrast with the hair at the back.

Stylist's note

It makes it easier if you remember you are working with three main sections; top, upper and lower back. Essentially you wrap the back sections across each other and bring the top over to join them.

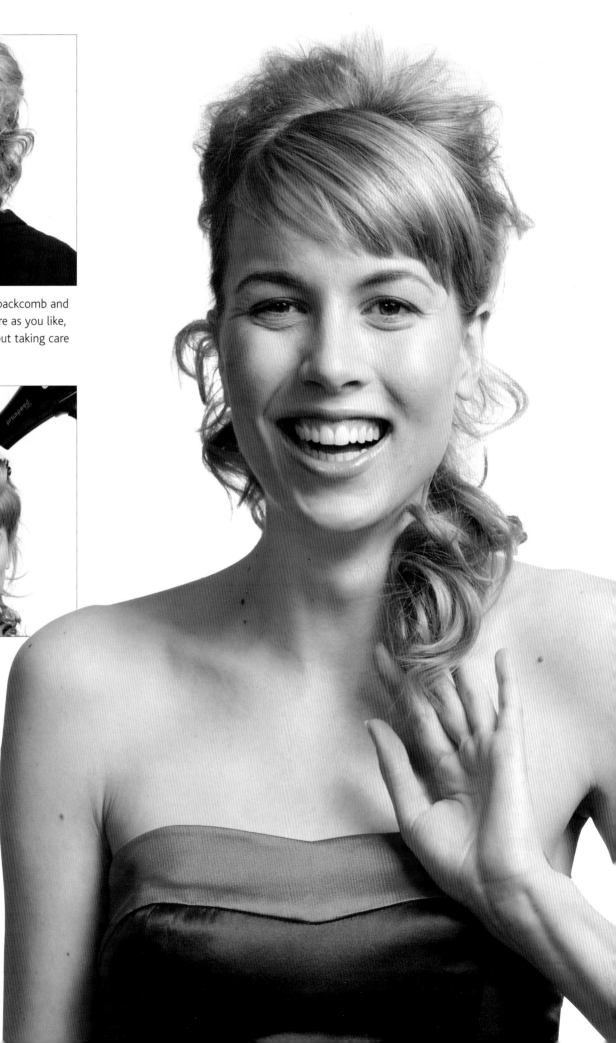

Creating a glamorous back-do

If you want to wear your hair down rather than up, but still be confident of having a style with a 'wow' factor, then this back-do is perfect. It draws hair off the face but still leaves some pieces around the neckline for softness.

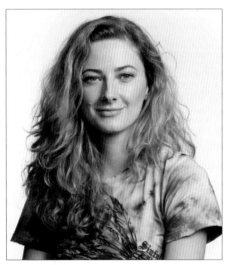

1 Brush dry hair and spritz with a styling spray.

2 Section your hair from the occipital area at the back of your head (leaving plenty of hair at the front and nape free) and draw the sectioned area into the centre back.

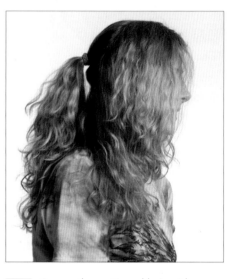

3 Secure the sectioned hair with a hairband (headband) to form a small ponytail.

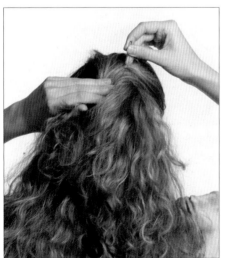

4 Draw the hair from one side at the front to cross the top of the base of the ponytail, and hold in place with an open-ended pin.

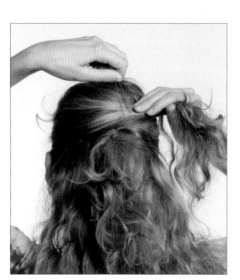

5 Repeat, drawing the hair from the other side to cross the top of the base of the ponytail, and hold in place with an open-ended pin.

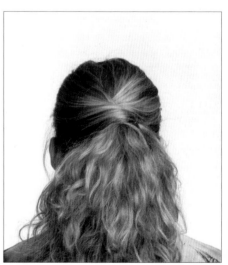

6 This is how your hair should look from the back.

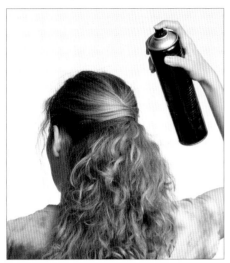

7 Spray with hairspray to hold.

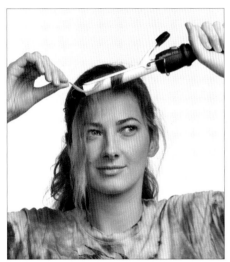

8 Curl any shorter, free front pieces with curling tongs for an individual touch, if you like.

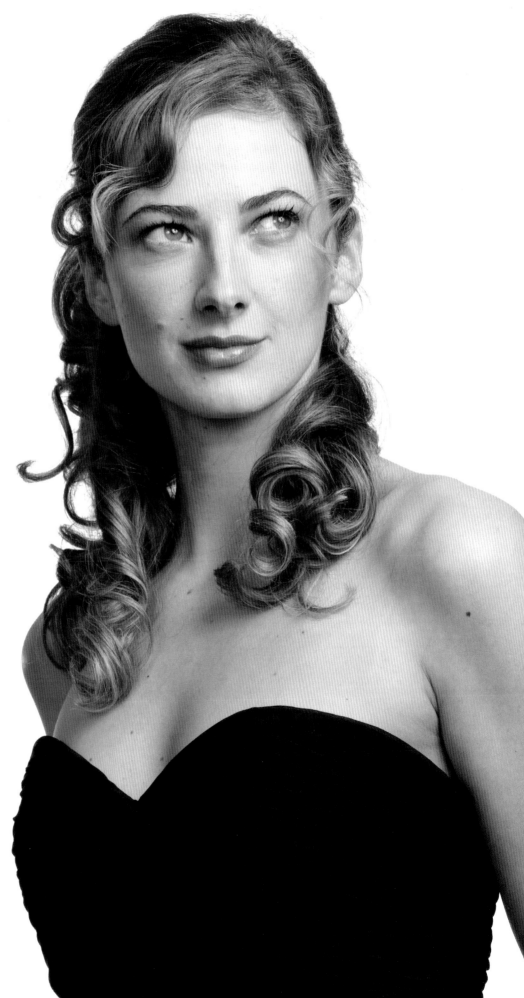

Stylist's note

This is a super-easy style that works well on curly or straight hair of mid- to long-length.

Creating a back-do with extra height

A really glamorous hairstyle needn't be fussy-looking or require you to set your hair first. This back-do is easy to achieve with just some pins and a hairbrush, and it looks fantastically elegant from the front, sides and back!

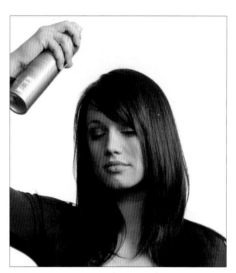

1 Brush clean, dry hair with a hairbrush to be completely tangle-free and smooth.

2 Spritz your hair all over with hairspray to add volume and to help with hold.

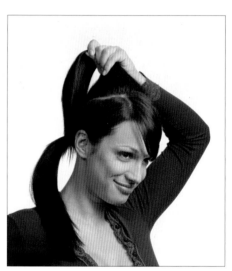

3 Section the top area of hair around the crown of your head and pin or tie the lower section out of the way with pins or hairbands (headbands). Here, the hair was put in a low ponytail.

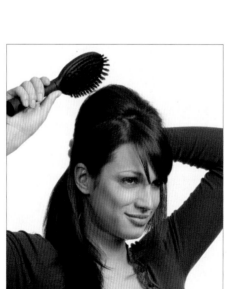

4 Working the free top area, back-brush the roots and mid lengths with a comb to create volume.

5 Using a flat brush, smooth over the very top layer of hair and draw it to the back of your head.

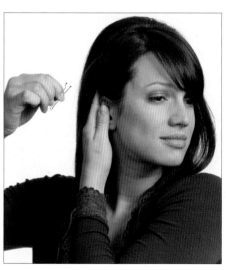

6 Undo the lower section that was previously pinned away, and brush through. Grip the hair at the sides for a flatter shape.

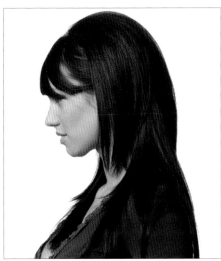

7 Your hair should now look like this, with height on the top of your head and smooth sides.

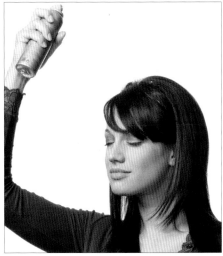

8 Spritz your hair with hairspray for hold and shine.

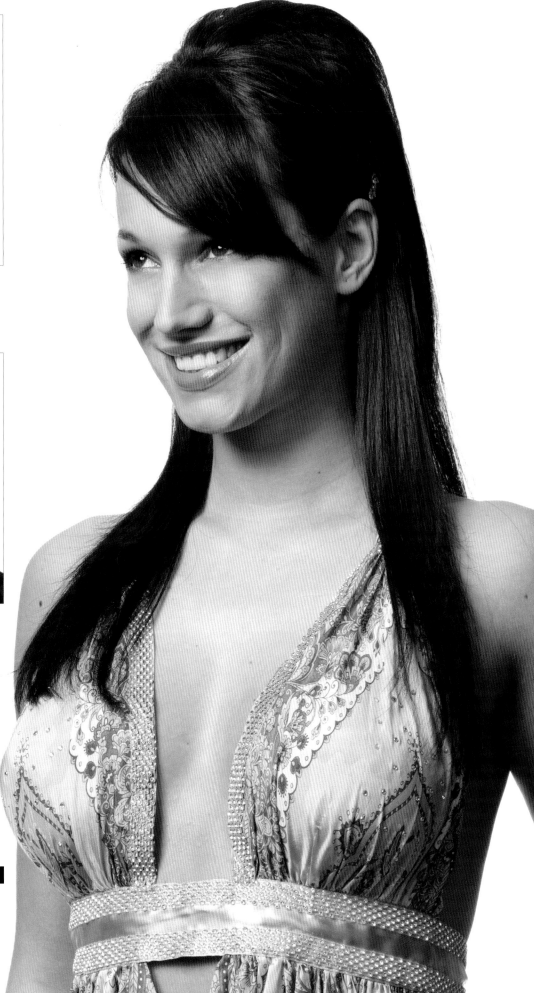

Stylist's note

Keep checking the side view to ensure you have a sense of height at the top back of your head for an elegant shape.

Creating an elegant top roll up-do

Choosing an up-do that adds height is a great way of appearing a little taller and more statuesque and often prompts you to stand that little bit straighter, too. It's all about conveying poise and elegance to create an impact.

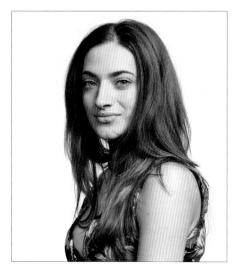

1 Brush dry hair to be completely tangle-free and smooth.

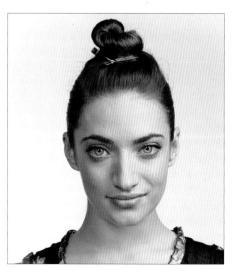

2 Section off the top area of hair and twist and clip it out of the way on top of your head.

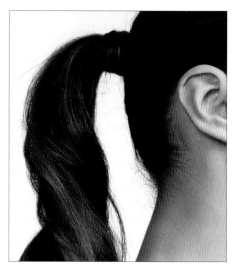

3 Draw your remaining hair to the centre back and secure in a reasonably tight ponytail. Wrap a section of hair around the hairband (headband) to conceal it.

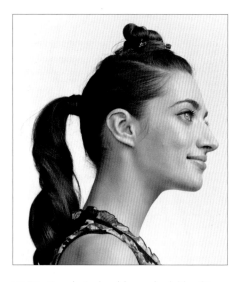

4 Your hair should now look like this.

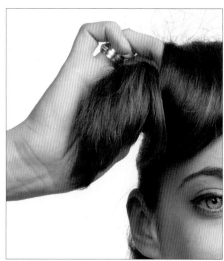

5 Unclip the top section of hair. Brush through then, using your hand to wrap the hair, start to form an upwards roll that adds height.

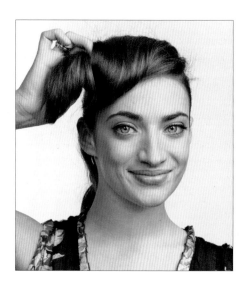

6 The roll should sit near the top front of your head. Tuck loose ends inside the roll to conceal them.

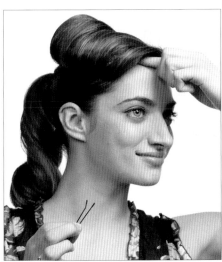

7 Hold the roll securely in place with extra-long hairgrips (bobby pins) by pushing them inside the roll so they don't show.

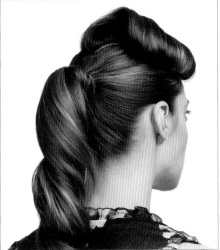

8 This is the back view of how the roll should look when you have finished. Spritz with hairspray for hold and shine.

Stylist's note

Once hair is pinned secure and sprayed, resist the temptation to fiddle with the style or keep touching it.

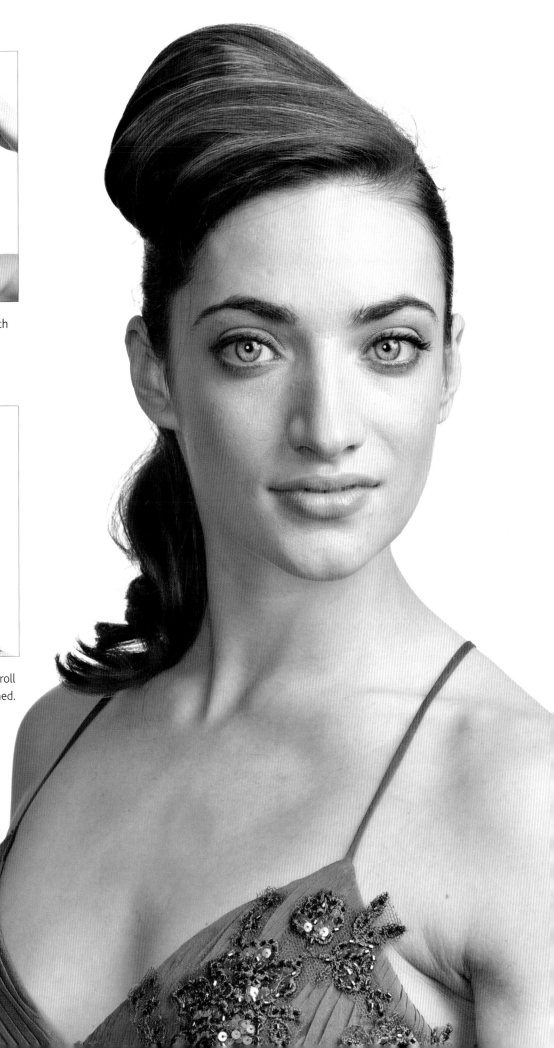

Creating an up-do with a front roll detail

This look is extremely elegant and is a real head-turner for a special occasion. Although it takes some time to do as it requires setting the hair before working the style, it is worth it in order to look and feel a million dollars!

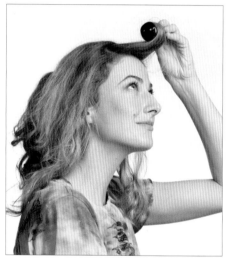

1 Spritz dry hair with styling lotion. Section it from ear to ear over the top of the head. Tie the back section in a ponytail with a hairband (headband).

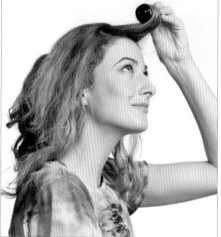

2 Place a heated roller in the front section of hair.

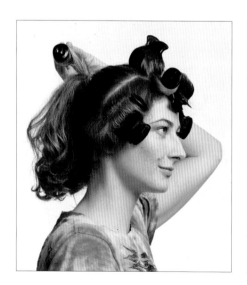

3 Place a second roller in the front, behind the first one, and one on each side (only use four in total in the front section to create waves rather than overt curl).

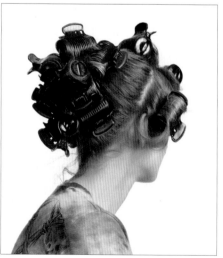

4 Place heated rollers in the ends of the ponytail too.

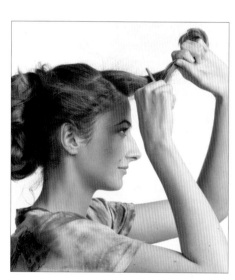

5 Continue in this way until all the hair is wrapped in heated rollers. Allow the rollers to cool completely before removing them.

6 Using a comb, backcomb the front section from roots to mid-lengths. Smooth over the top layer of hair.

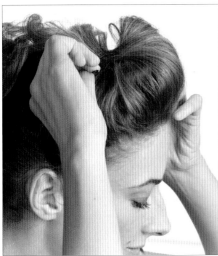

7 Wrapping the hair around your hand, roll this front section towards the back of your head and grip in place.

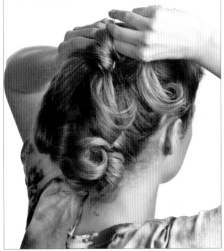

8 Without brushing through, take sections of the ponytail and grip them in loops over the base of the ponytail until they are all gripped in place. Spritz with hairspray to hold.

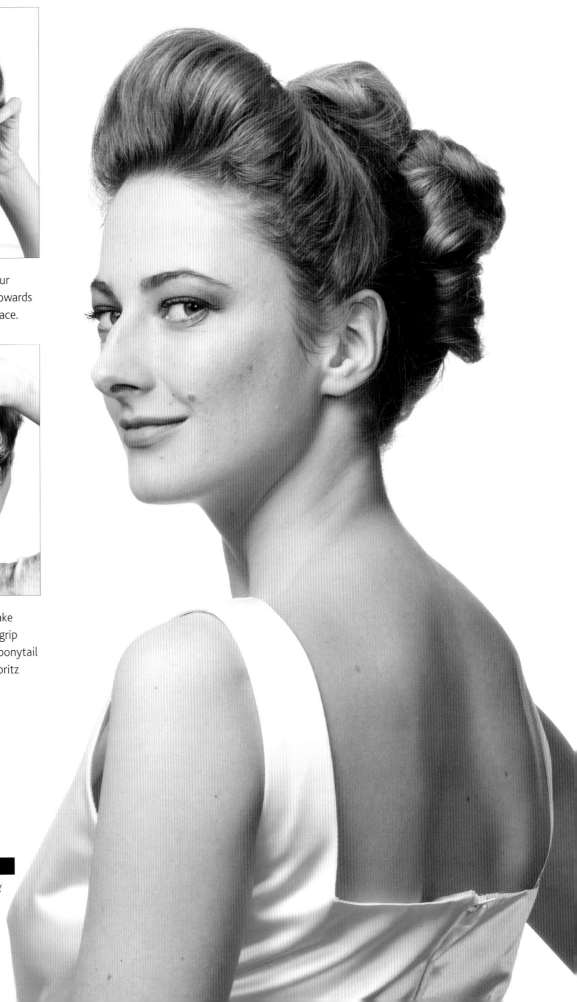

Stylist's notes

Do practise this style before your big day to build confidence, as it is moderately difficult to create.

Creating a chic, tonged tumbling up-do

This fantastic up-do makes a stunning special look that balances a smooth groomed front view with a glorious cascade of hair at the back. It's the perfect complement for a chic evening gown – red carpet hair made easy!

You will need
- Sectioning clips
- Hairband
- Small-barrelled curling tongs
- Hairspray
- Bristle brush
- Pins
- Open-ended pins

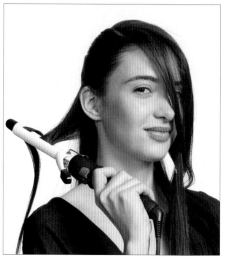

1 Section dry hair to form a front piece, side sections and a back section, which is secured in a high ponytail with a hairband (headband) at the back of the head in the middle.

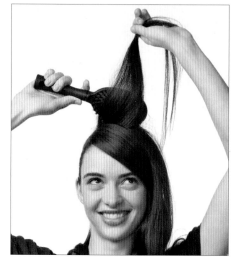

2 Hang the front section across your face, then wrap small sections of loose hair everywhere else round small-barrelled curling tongs to form ringlets.

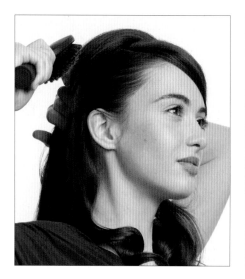

3 Spritz hair with hairspray to add volume and guts. Tuck the smooth front piece behind one ear so it is out of the way. Take hair from the top section and backbrush at the roots using a bristle brush.

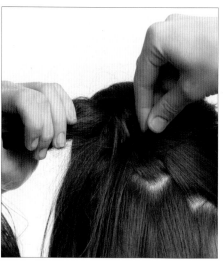

4 Smooth this backbrushed top section over with a bristle brush and draw it to the back of the head.

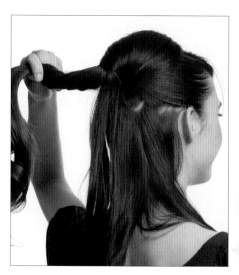

5 Wrap this top section hair round the base of the high ponytail to conceal the hairband and pin in place.

6 Lift the free ends of the ponytail with one hand and twist loosely.

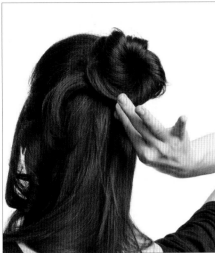

7 Wrap the twist round near the base of the ponytail and pin in place, forming a loose bun shape.

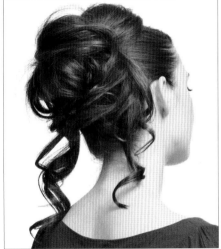

8 Pin up all free hair, including the front piece previously tucked behind the ear, around the bun, using open-ended pins to secure, and building up the shape of the bun. Spritz with hairspray to hold.

Stylist's notes

Don't worry about making the back view look too neat. As long as curls are well-defined, pinning them up randomly is fine.

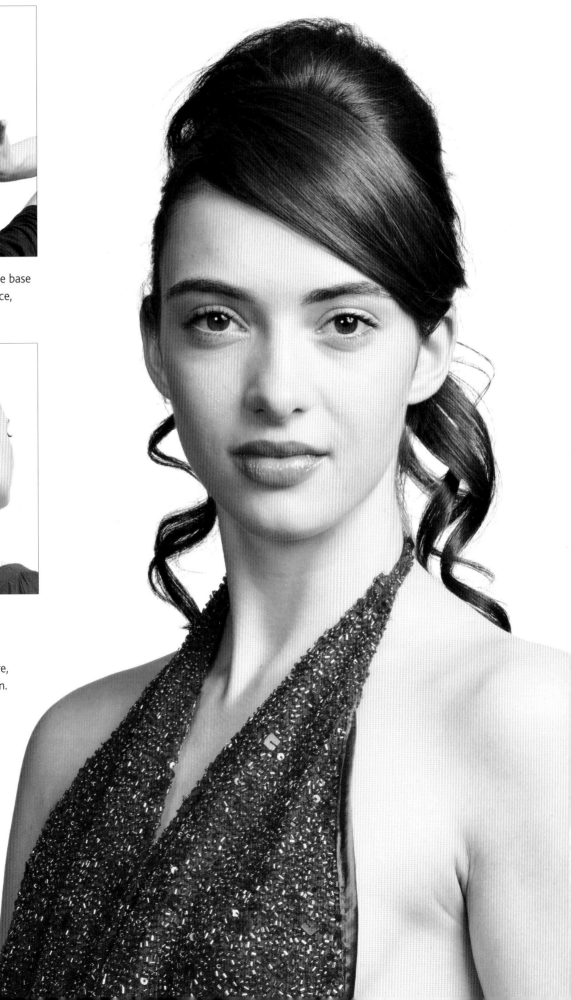

Creating an up-do on curly hair

A mass of natural curls can be a real asset when creating an up-do as you already have movement and texture to build up a fantastic shape. The curls also provide softness around the face and look really adorable.

You will need
- Moisture crème or defining paste
- Hairgrips (bobby pins)
- Hairspray
- Accessory (optional)

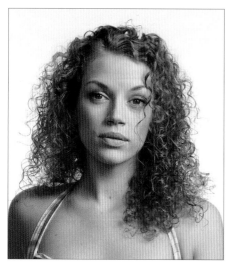

1 Allow dry hair to hang naturally without brushing it or trying to smooth it out.

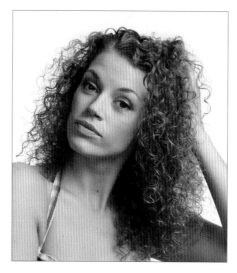

2 Put a small amount of moisture crème or defining paste into the palm of one hand, then rub your hands together and apply it to your hair with your fingers to define your curls.

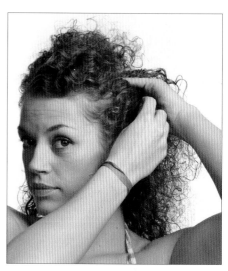

3 Use hairgrips (bobby pins) to pin up lower sections of hair to create shape and add height.

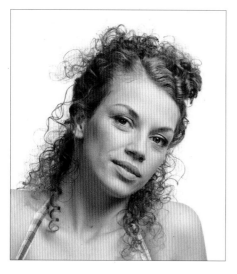

4 This could now be a finished look for a less dressy occasion.

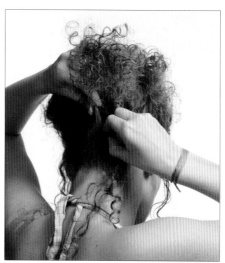

5 Alternatively, continue to pin up more sections of hair for a more dramatic up-do.

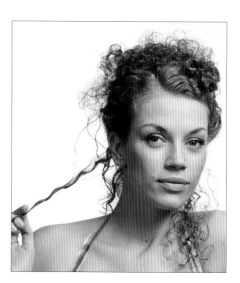

6 Loosen small pieces of hair to frame your face and soften the look.

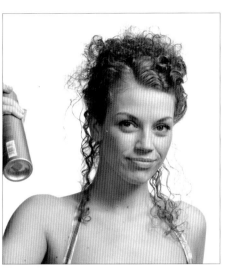

7 Spray your hair liberally with hairspray to hold.

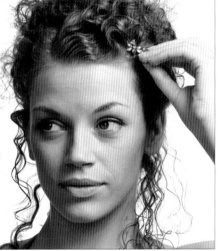

8 Add an accessory to suit the occasion, if you like.

Stylist's note

Sparingly apply a crème or paste to encourage the curls to sit more evenly and retain their natural shape.

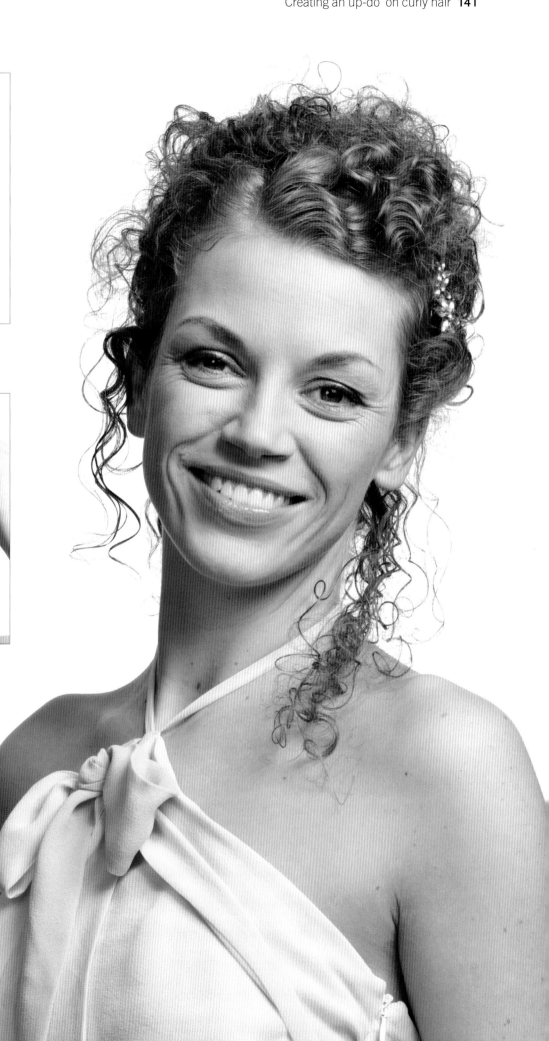

Creating an up-do on crimped hair

The crimping detail in this technique adds a really interesting texture to the hair. Also, by crimping hair before you put it up into a style, you will add body so that hairgrips stay put and there is added volume and shape to work with.

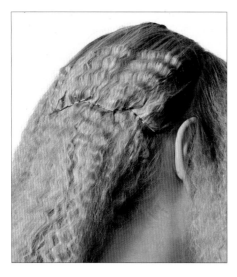

1 Section crimped, long hair from ear to ear. Working the back section, place hairgrips (bobby pins) criss-crossed just below the occipital bone.

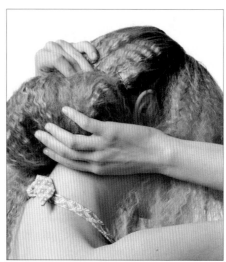

2 Taking all the hair from below the line of crossed hairgrips, roll it outwards from the ends up and pin it in place over the crossed hairgrips using open-ended pins.

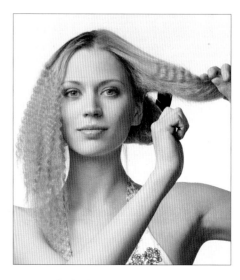

3 Lift the hair from the side-front (previously left free) on one side and backcomb the roots with a dressing-out brush or a comb.

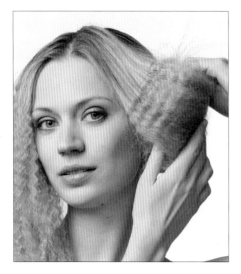

4 Wrap this backcombed hair outwards and backwards to form a barrel shape.

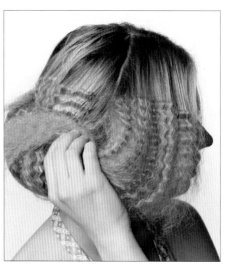

5 Grip the wrapped hair behind the ear and tuck in any ends to blend with the back roll formed earlier.

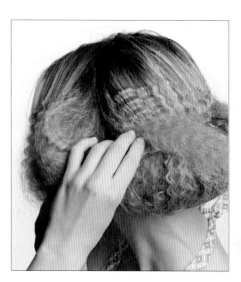

6 Repeat the process of backcombing and rolling on the other side with the remaining loose hair.

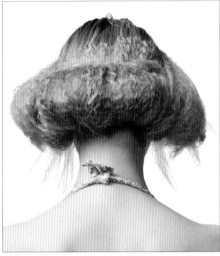

7 This is how the back of your head should now look.

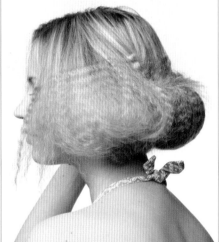

8 Spritz your hair all over with hairspray for hold. Don't worry if pieces of hair fly free at the front, it helps to soften the outline.

Stylist's notes

This style is stunning but quite complex so ask a friend to help – or position lots of mirrors around you so you can see what you are doing.

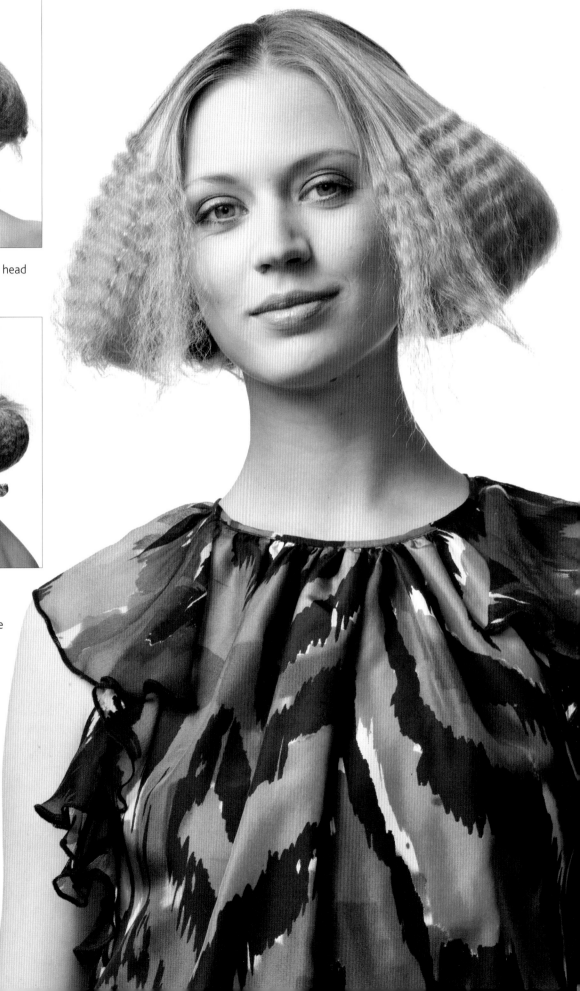

Creating a loose wedding style

If you want to wear a tiara or a very striking headdress in your hair, it may be best to wear your hair in a loose style. It's important to place the headpiece far enough forward that it will show clearly in photographs.

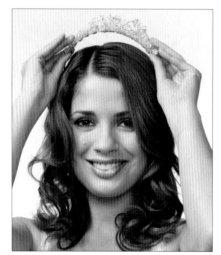

Stylist's note

Always try on a headdress before you buy it to ensure it sits comfortably on your head shape. Check if it's possible to bend it slightly so it fits your head perfectly.

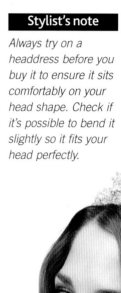

1 Create loose curls on your hair by spritzing through clean, dry hair with heat-protective spray then using curling tongs on the hair or setting it on large heated rollers.

2 If necessary, spritz your hair with hairspray for hold, then position the headdress on the very top of your head to sit just behind your ears.

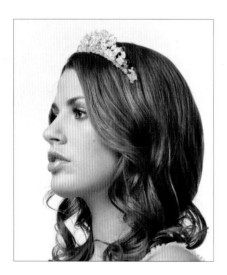

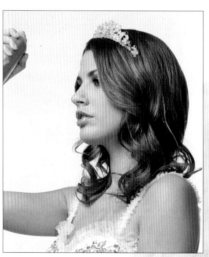

3 Ensure the headdress is not dragging your hair back from the sides; you should be placing the headdress in the hair as it falls naturally, not using it as a headband.

4 Spritz your hair all over with shine spray to finish.

Creating a stylish wedding back-do

For an elegant style that works well with a veil without looking too traditional, then this side-do is perfect. Providing an offset point to fix the veil for a ceremony, it looks equally chic from all angles once the veil is removed.

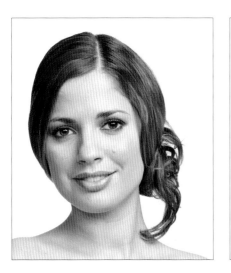

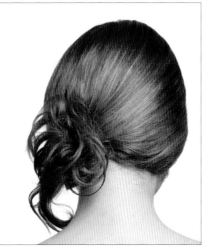

Stylist's note

Once you have removed the veil, try fixing a new hair ornament in its place, if you like.

1 Set your hair in large heated rollers to create loose curls. Brush these lightly and sweep to one side of your head. Twist the hair once and grip in place with hairgrips (bobby pins).

2 This is how the back should look. Spritz the hair with hairspray to hold and calm any flyaway hairs.

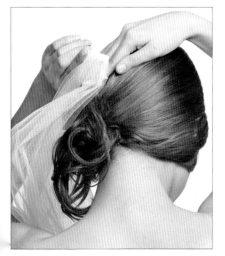

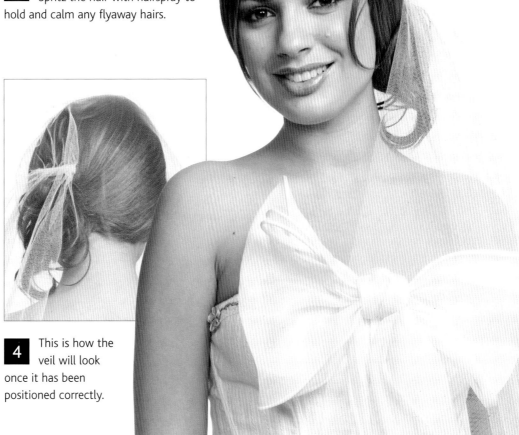

3 Place a veil to grip at the base of the twist where there is enough body and texture to secure it properly.

4 This is how the veil will look once it has been positioned correctly.

Creating a contemporary wedding back-do

For an individual touch, go for an asymmetric look with this side style that works brilliantly with larger or more striking flowers or hair ornaments. It's a fabulous take on a classic technique and will make your wedding day that little bit extra special.

You will need

- Bristle brush
- Hairgrips (bobby pins)
- Flowers or hair ornaments
- Open-ended pins
- Hairspray

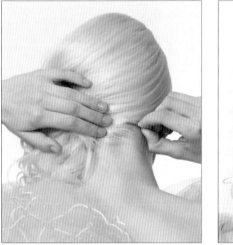

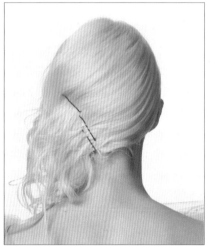

Stylist's note

To create a little bit of height, try backcombing the roots of the top section before smoothing it over and drawing all the hair to the side.

1 Brush curled hair to be smooth and tangle-free. Using a bristle brush, gently sweep your hair to one side and hold in place with your hand.

2 Place hairgrips (bobby pins) in a line, as pictured here, to hold the hair in place (use grips to match your hair colour — these are dark for illustrative purposes).

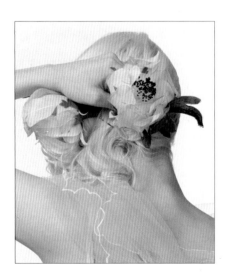

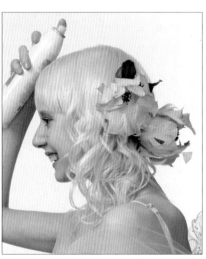

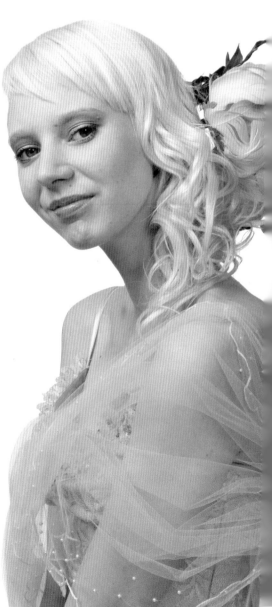

3 Fix flowers or other hair ornaments at the back using open-ended pins to disguise where the hair is already gripped.

4 Spritz your hair liberally with hairspray for hold.

Creating a classic wedding back-do

This look is so effortlessly simple and yet perfect for that fresh, classic feel. It's all about creating a delightful shape that balances and complements the intricate detail of the wedding dress and hair ornament.

You will need

- Curling tongs
- Hair ornament
- Hairgrips (bobby pins)
- Hairspray
- Shine spray

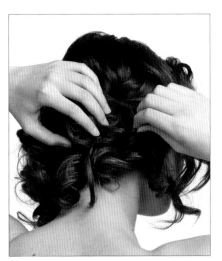

1 Tong clean, dry hair to add waves or very loose curls. The look is natural and romantic without being too over-done.

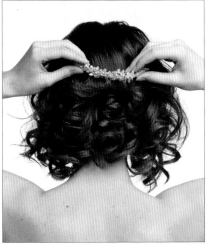

2 Position the hair ornament (in this case a comb) just below the middle at the back of the head. Check in a mirror that you are happy with its placement and that it is secure.

Stylist's note

Choose a hair ornament that is affixed to your hair with a deep comb for added security.

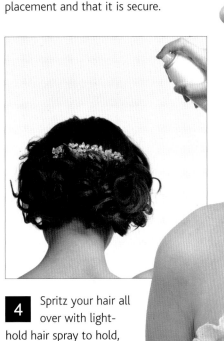

3 Lift sections from the bottom of your hair and pin them up securely underneath the hair ornament to create shape.

4 Spritz your hair all over with light-hold hair spray to hold, then shine spray to finish.

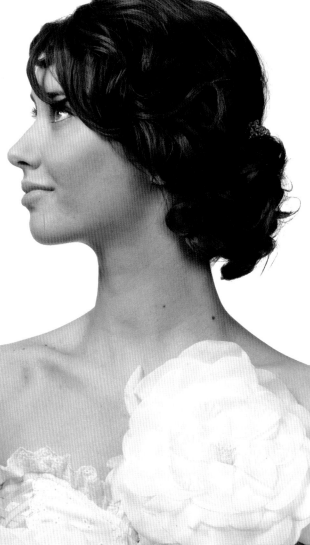

Creating a romantic wedding pin-up

Keeping a real romanticism in the hair with plenty of curl detail, this up-do is sweet and beautiful without being too intricate to complete. Place flowers wherever you like at the back – the roses here work well with the softness of the curl.

You will need
- Heat-protective spray
- Curling tongs or heated rollers
- Hairgrips (bobby pins)
- Strong-hold hairspray
- Hair ornaments

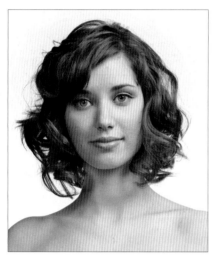

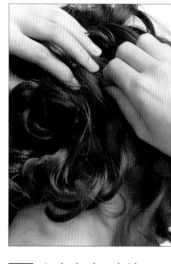

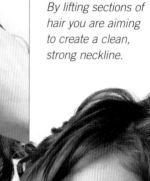

Stylist's note

By lifting sections of hair you are aiming to create a clean, strong neckline.

1 Create loose curls on your hair by spritzing through clean, dry hair with heat-protective spray, then wrapping hair in curling tongs or setting it on large heated rollers.

2 At the back and sides, create an elegant shape by taking random sections of hair and gripping them up. Leave some tendrils free around your face.

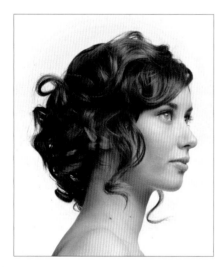

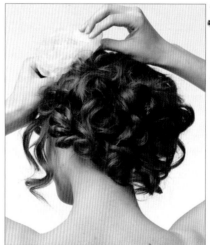

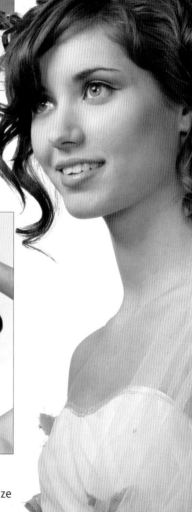

3 Pin the pieces of hair off the neck as this gives a stronger line to the look that contrasts well with the loose tendrils at the front.

4 Spritz your hair all over with strong-hold hairspray. Accessorize the up-do with flowers if you like, to complement the dress and romantic mood of the style.

Creating a chic wedding up-do

For an ultra-sleek line that is superbly elegant and sophisticated, consider a classic chignon. The simple, clean shape of the hairstyle will help the veil to lie in a lovely cascading fall of fabric and it will also look good once you remove it.

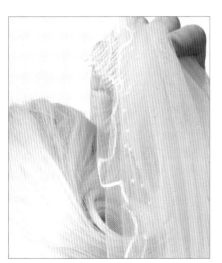

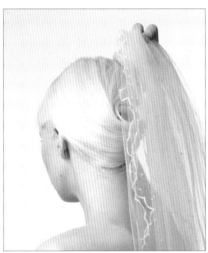

Stylist's note

Wherever you style the chignon to sit will be where you need to fix the veil, so keep an eye on your profile to see which position looks best.

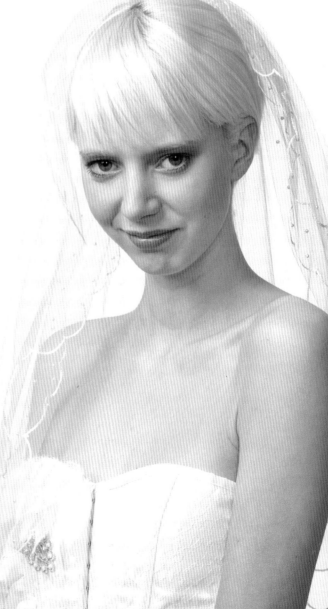

1 Form clean, dry hair into a chignon (see pages 122–3). Spritz with light-hold hairspray and shine spray to finish.

2 Position the top of the veil over the top of the chignon, holding it by the comb, so that the comb attachment is fixed above the coil at the top of the chignon.

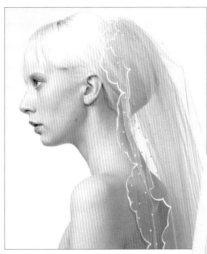

3 This is how the top of the chignon should look.

4 Push the comb fixing the veil in place so the veil hangs over the top of the chignon. This is the side view of how it should look.

Wearing a hat

It has been a long time since it was de rigeur for women to wear them, but hats are still a great way of finishing an outfit to look really formal, enormously stylish or simply individual. The trick is in knowing what hat shape suits you and exactly how to wear it.

Apart from grabbing a woolly hat to keep warm in winter, many people only wear a hat on a special occasion and so can feel a bit overwhelmed by the choice on offer. It can be a daunting prospect to find a hat to suit an outfit, event, and hairstyle, but life will be made easier if you figure out several factors in advance:

- Will you be keeping your hat on for much of the time, or do you need a hairstyle that will work once the hat is removed and won't be flattened?
- Does your hat need to be practical in any way – such as providing shade for your eyes, or staying put in inclement weather – or is the hat only ornamental?
- Fix your outfit first, then find a hat, not the other way around. If you feel confident in your clothes, then you'll have more confidence with the hat.

- Remember, you can either wear a hat to complete a look, or you can choose one to be the focal point. The key is not to choose a hat to fight with your outfit – only one will be the winner, the other a sinner!

Proportion and balance

The art of wearing a hat to stunning effect lies in understanding proportion and balance and choosing a size and shape accordingly. A hat can look fabulous on the stand, but that doesn't mean it will necessarily look as good on you, and it's not just a question of how it fits. For example, big hats can swamp petite faces and bodies, or even look like you've got a halo. A small hat might look totally wrong with your hairstyle and maybe even draw attention to your least flattering features.

Equally, the right hat can be worn the wrong way; perhaps too far back, or tilted in an unbecoming way that ruins the overall effect. Here's a simple guide to scale and shape, together with pointers on what works best:

- A large hat will swamp a small face, and if worn with a voluminous outfit, can end up looking rather comical. Instead, wear something that opens up your face, with a small or no brim.
- A cloche or brimless hat can accentuate a round face, and small or close-fitting hats can make a round face look bigger. Choose dynamic shapes and asymmetric lines instead.
- A tall hat on a long face only serves to make you look even more drawn out. Opt for less height and perhaps more width to balance the look.

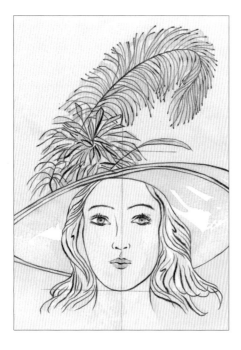

Above *A hat with width balances a long face shape. Wearing it with some hair or part of the hat coming across the forehead will enhance the shortening effect.*

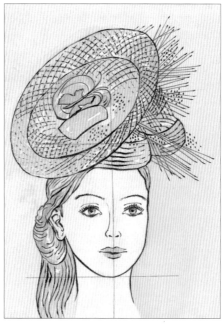

Above *A round face needs some height and structure to help balance it. Wearing a hat at an angle also serves to vary the line for a more flattering look.*

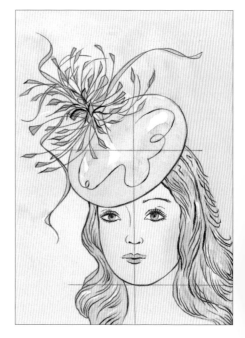

Above *Wearing a hat (or fascinator) to one side and low over the face is a great way to balance a strong square face shape and is a look that is intriguing and timeless.*

- A wide-brimmed hat on a heart-shaped face can simply make your chin disappear, whereas a hat with an asymmetrical or upswept brim can draw attention to the eyes.
- Rather than try a hat, you can opt for a fascinator (a large ornament), which is ideal for small face shapes or for wearing all day long, from a wedding ceremony to a reception perhaps.

How to wear a hat

A hat is supposed to be worn at an angle to follow the contours of your head; so it works with the outline shape. The result of this is that the hat appears to be a natural extension of your face rather than something that looks like it's following you around and irritating you.

Think of your face and head in four quarters and follow the rules illustrated below. You will first need to decide on your face shape.

Tip

When using feathers or ornaments to create a headpiece, the secret is in choosing something with a line that follows the curve of the head. It's much more elegant.

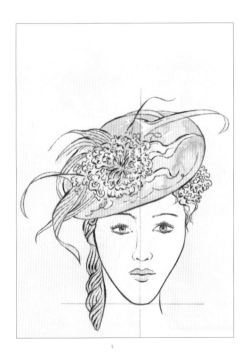

Above *A petite face can be swamped by a large hat, so choose smaller ones and wear them to one side. Details such as veils or ornaments add width for balance and shape.*

How to make and wear a headpiece

If you can't find the exact hat you want, then how about making your own headpiece or fascinator, which does the job without costing a fortune, and works for indoors or out. You can adapt this method to a variety of flowers or other ornaments.

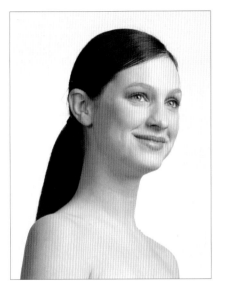

1 Draw hair into a ponytail at the back of the head, fixing it fairly low at the nape and making it as smooth as possible, applying a light gel if required. Calm any flyaways with some hairspray.

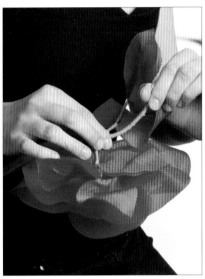

2 Take a large fabric flower and bend the wired stem to curve into a half-moon shape that fits the curve of your head. This way it will be more comfortable when it is fixed in place.

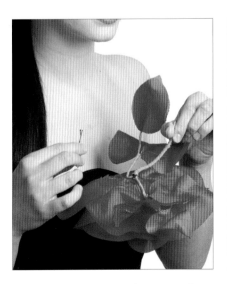

3 Use several grips (bobby pins) that fit around the stem to create a way of fixing it to your hair. Try and match these grips to your hair colour to disguise them once they are in place.

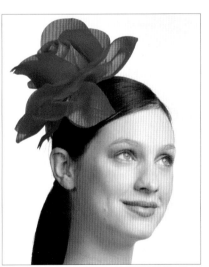

4 Place the flower where it best balances your face shape, and complements the outfit. Fix it in place, crossing grips for security, and arrange petals to cover the grips. Spray for hold.

Formal hats

Wearing a striking hat or headpiece usually means you don't need a complicated hairstyle or up-do.

1 An ornate, asymmetric hat worn with a clean, smooth offset ponytail provides dramatic shape that will make a real impact. The point is that this hat works best with a neat hairstyle where hair is swept clear off the face and shoulders for a defined neckline.

2 A large-brimmed picture hat looks fantastic set squarely on the head to contrast with loose, soft hair. It also complements the simple line of the dress. The trick is to wear the hat straight so the brim dips across the forehead slightly.

3 The more decorative the hat, the more you need clean lines in the hairstyle and shape of the clothing; it's important that nothing fights for attention. A hat with height is best avoided if you have a long face. Here, the soft cream is the perfect contrast for a dark hair colouring.

4 A headpiece (sometimes called a fascinator) rather than a hat can be very striking. Here, wearing a headpiece to one side perfectly balances the asymmetric, one-shoulder line of the dress. (It would not work if it were set to the other side of the head, however).

5 The soft feathering detailing of this disc-shaped hat is mirrored beautifully by the soft, gentle curls of the hairstyle and balances the unfussy line of the dress. Having the hat forward on the forehead adds height to a round or square face.

6 A very simple, smooth blow-dried hairstyle is just right for balancing the intricate styling of this dress and the bow detailing of this headpiece. Having a headpiece with the ornamentation to one side adds interest and individuality so the look is not overly demure.

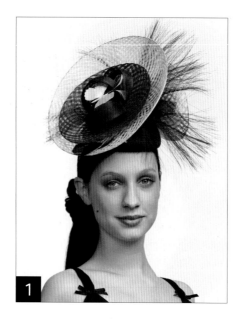

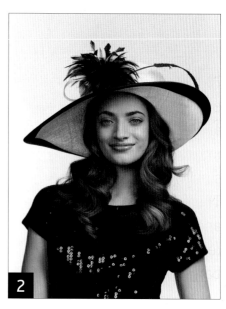

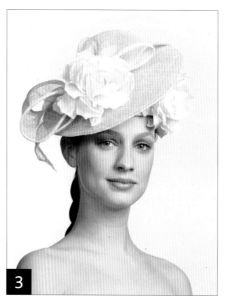

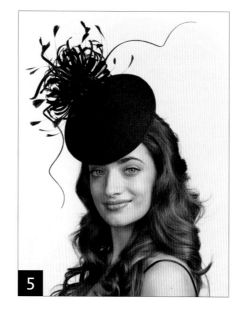

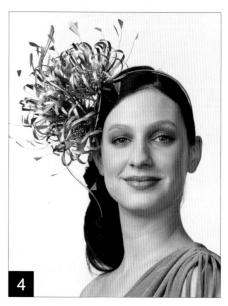

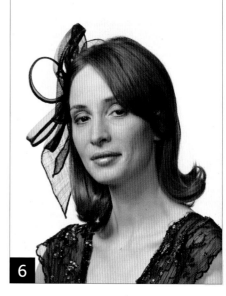

Informal hats

Hats are extremely useful for everyday wear, whether they are used to keep you warm, to shade you from the sun, or simply as a fashion statement. There are many different types and styles, but the same rules regarding proportion and balance apply as for formal hats.

1 A peaked cap not only looks good, but has a dual function as it keeps your head warm while shading your eyes from low winter sun. Leave some hair showing to avoid looking too masculine.

2 Woolly hats are perfect for skiing holidays, and help protect your hair from reflected sunlight bouncing off the snow as well as keeping you warm.

3 Sun hats come in many different sizes, so try on several types, from large or floppy to more rigid or structured. It is important they have a brim to offer protection to both skin and eyes.

4 Floppy knitted hats are best worn further back on the head.

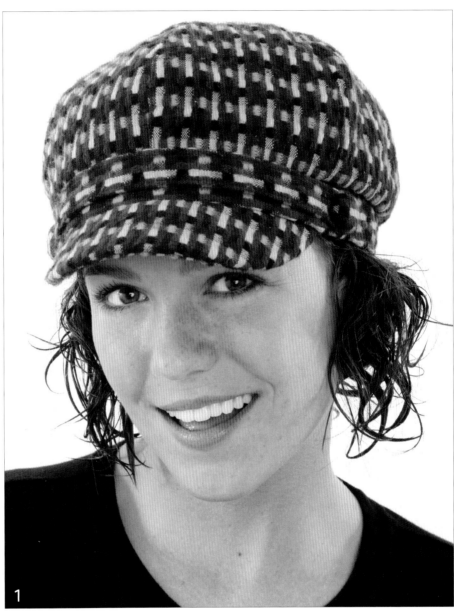

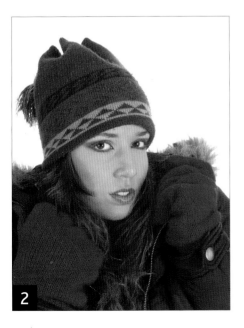

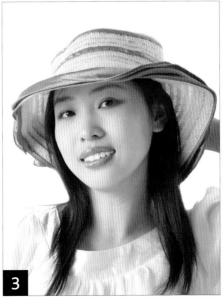

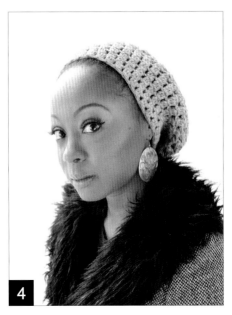

Choosing accessories

Use hair accessories to instantly enhance a simple hairstyle, or completely change your look. Drawing hair off the face in a hairband or clipping a section of hair to one side with a decorative slide or clip is a neat, fast way to switch styles.

Today's wealth of decorative accessories such as beaded, jewelled, feathered and ribboned headbands, hairbands (headbands), hairgrips (bobby pins) and hair slides (barrettes) mean there is no need to be plain and utilitarian. To help you choose, here are a few top tips:

▪ Is the accessory to be simply decorative or does it need to hold hair firmly in place? Make sure it will be up to the job.

▪ It can be a mistake to select accessories in colours that exactly match your clothes, bags or shoes – the overall effect will be a little too cutey pie! Unless that's a look you like, of course.

▪ For jewelled accessories, less can often be more. If you have high-impact ornaments in your hair, tone down the rest of your jewellery and wear a simple, one-colour top.

▪ Some accessories, such as headbands and ribbons, are so much associated with schoolgirl looks that you need to be careful to select fabrics and shapes that reflect your personal style today. Velvets, sumptuous satin and grown-up patterns will help.

Below Jewelled hairgrips, slides and pins don't need to be large – small ones will still catch the light beautifully.

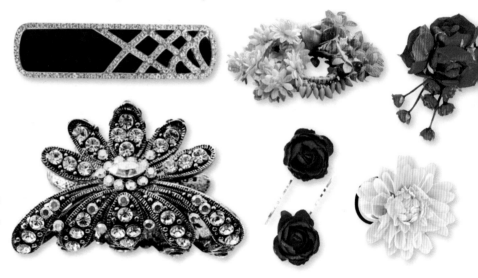

Above Diamanté clips and slides are very striking, especially in a simple hairstyle, and are best worn with understated jewellery.

▪ Do experiment at home to be sure you are comfortable before wearing anything adventurous, quirky or particularly dynamic – there's nothing worse than going out and not feeling confident.

▪ Don't assume accessories are for long hair only. A hair clip or pin in short hair can be fun, glamorous or sophisticated. Just remember that understated can be the best way to start.

▪ Fast fixes include hair clips or pins placed where there is an interesting detail

Above Flowers have a timeless appeal and there are some really fantastic designs available, from sophisticated to fun.

in the hair to draw attention to, perhaps at the base of a bun or ponytail.

▪ Tiaras and headbands look good on any length hair but need to be positioned properly: straight across the forehead; high at the base of an up-do; or on long hair in a direct line from ear to ear over the very top of the head.

▪ Use jewellery to make your own customized accessories. Bracelets can be fixed using hairgrips (bobby pins) pushed through the chain and brooches can be glued on to hair slides or hair clips. You could wrap wire round the ornament and attach to hair slides, hairgrips or combs.

▪ Newly-washed hair can be too slippery for accessories to stay in. Spritz hair with hairspray to add guts, or even backcomb the roots slightly.

▪ Remember heavy accessories can drag down or fall out, so don't be too ambitious.

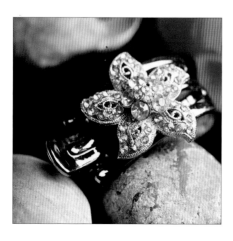

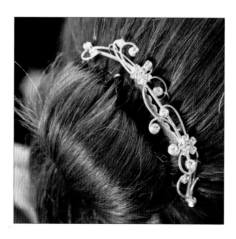

Left Work out in advance whether the accessory will need to hold hair in place or whether it is purely decorative, as here.

Flowers

For special occasions such as weddings, fresh flowers are perfect, but these days there are so many fantastic fabric flowers available that you can look fabulous without fear of your hairpiece wilting.

1 A large flower worn to one side is all the ornamentation this soft, curly hairstyle needs. Place the flower above the ear on the opposite side to where hair is swept (i.e. the same side as a parting).

2 Fabric flowers on bands or gripped to one side of the base of a ponytail are very striking. The longer your hair, the larger the flower should be to prevent it looking too indistinct.

3 Place a flower at the base of a bun for a simple, effective detail. Having the flower to one side or slightly below the top of the bun is more elegant than placing it above the bun.

4 An exaggerated flower adds drama to a ponytail. The larger and more ornate the flower, the more clean and sleek the hairstyle and clothing need to be.

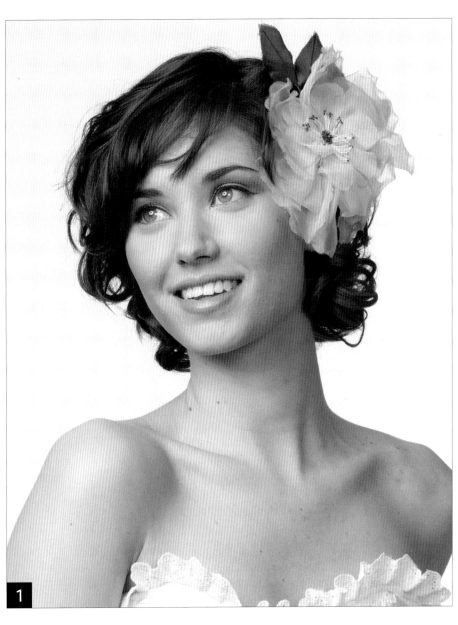

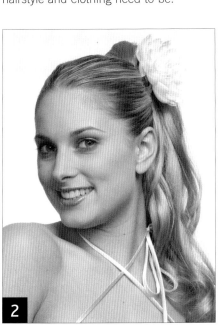

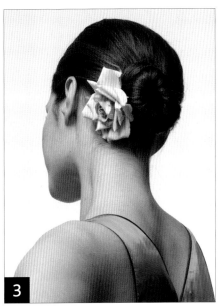

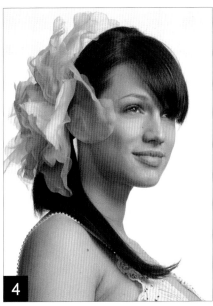

Hairgrips and hair slides

Ornamental hairgrips, hair clips, hair pins and hair slides can be a subtle way to draw the eye to a detail in the hairstyle, without being too high impact. Choose a colour that complements your hair tone and your outfit.

1 Two matching hair slides (barrettes) can be pinned to the swirl detail of a simple up-do to lend it an elegant touch for a special occasion.

2 Here a pair of elegant shell-shaped pins contrast with the curl in the hair and emphasize the twist.

3 Highly decorative hair slides add glamour to a pretty hair style, and are especially useful for weddings or other special occasions.

4 Even small, pretty hairgrips (bobby pins) can make a statement. Here, the subtle sparkle finishes the style perfectly.

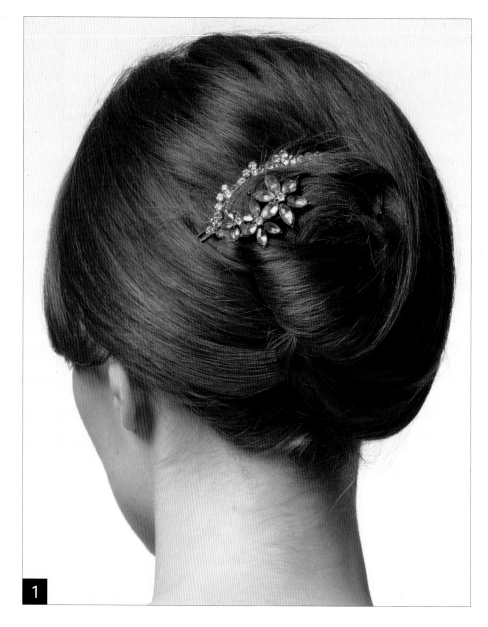

1

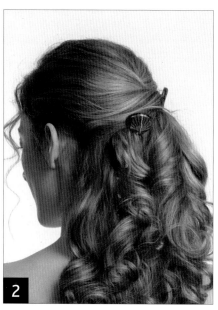

2

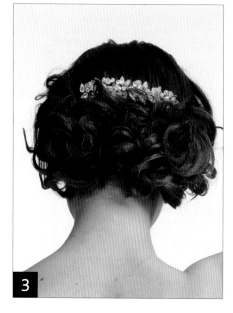

3

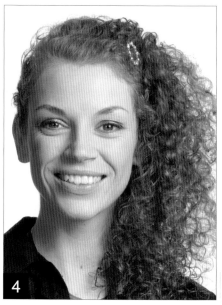

4

Bows and ribbons

There is a wide range of bows on offer, from tailored to floppy, and they often come ready-tied and attached to hair clips or hair slides. You could also simply form them yourself from ribbons or fabric that matches or contrasts with your outfit.

1 Most ribbons, especially those made from silk or satin fabric, will be too slippery to hold hair in place, so wrap them over a hairband (headband).

2 Adding a neat, ready-made bow lifts a simple ponytail in an understated way. It is smart enough for most formal occasions or can be worn for a night out.

3 Try winding a ribbon round a long section of hair and finishing with a loose bow for a different look.

4 Decorative bows can be attached to hair slides (barrettes) or hair clips, and add interest to a simple, neat style.

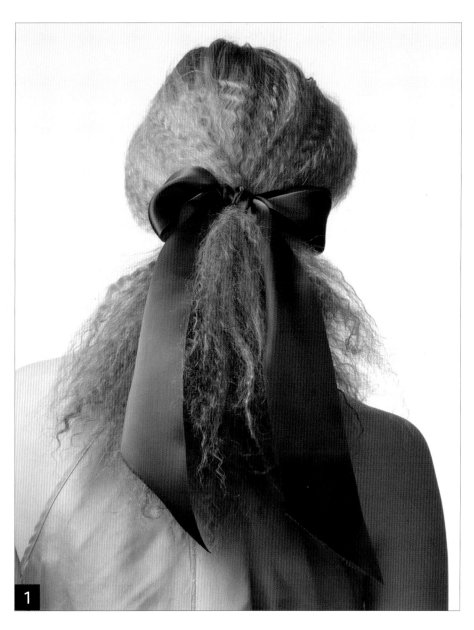

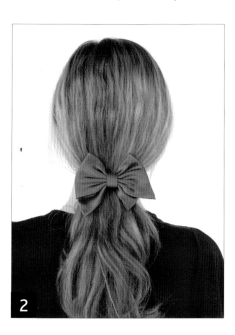

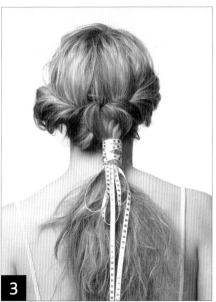

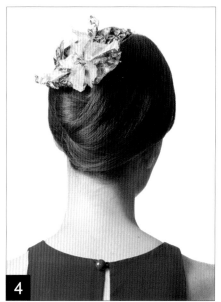

Index

Figures in italics indicate captions.

accessories 154
added hair 19, 77–83

back-dos
   Creating a Back-do with Extra Height
      132–3
   Creating a Classic Wedding Back-do 147
   Creating a Contemporary Wedding
      Back-do 146
   Creating a Glamorous Back-do 130–1
   Creating a Mussed-up Back-do on
      Mid-length Hair 128–9
   Creating a Sweet Asymmetric
      Back-do 100–1
   Creating a Stylish Wedding Back-do 145
bangs *see* fringe
bendable rods 13, *13,* 66–7
blow-drying 22, 23, 24, 25, 26–7, 28–9,
      30–1, 32, 33, 34, 35, 36, 37, 38, 39,
      40–1, 42–3, 44–5, 46
bobby pins *see* hairgrips
bobs 26–7
bows *154,* 157
braids *see* plaits
buns
   Creating a Perfect Ballerina Bun 92–3
   Creating a Perfect Woven Bun 96–7
   Creating a Slick Offset Ballerina Bun
      120–1
   Creating a Twist Back-do on Mid-length
      Hair 126

chemical processing 19
chignons
   Creating a Perfect Classic Chignon
      122–3
   Creating a Perfect French Roll 94–5
combs 12, *12*
conditioning sprays/creams 17
creams 17
crèmes, styling 16
crimping
   Creating an Up-do on Crimped Hair
      142–3
   Crimping Dressed Hair for Partial
      Texture 62
   Crimping Loose Hair for a Random
      Texture Effect 63

Crimping Loose Hair for All-over
      Texture 60–1
curl-activators 16
curling
   Creating Sumptuous Curls on
      Straight Hair 116–17
   Using Barrel Curls to Create Volume
      and Soft Curl 69
   Using Bendable Rods to Create an
      Even Curl 66–7
   Using Pin-curls to Create a Gentle,
      Tumbling Curl 68
   Using Tongs for Different Curled
      Effects 48–9
   Using Tongs to Create All-over Curl 51
   Using Tongs to Create Random Spiral
      Curls 50
curly hair
   Blow-drying Curly Hair for a Soft,
      Smooth Look 44–5
   Creating a Glamorous Pin-up on
      Shorter Curly Hair 107
   Creating a Quick Party Look on Curly
      Hair 112–13
   Creating an Up-do on Curly Hair 140–1

dressing hair 19
drying techniques 18

extensions 19

fine hair 10
finger-drying 18
French pleat
   Creating a Perfect French Pleat 98–9
French roll
   Creating a Perfect French Roll 94–5
fringes: A Range of Fringe Finishes for
      Different Effects 84–5
   Blow-drying to Add Emphasis to a
      Deep, Wide Fringe 46
   Fitting and Wearing a False Fringe 81
   Fitting and Wearing a Wig with a
      Natural Hair Fringe 77

gel
   Using Gel to Create a Smooth, Wet
      Look on Shorter Hair 74
   Using Gel to Create Spikes on Shorter
      Hair 75

hair balms 16
hair clips 12, *12,* 154, 156
hair pins 12, *12,* 154, *154,* 156
hair slides 154, *154,* 156
hairbrushes 10–11, *10, 11*
hairdryers 14, *14*
hairgrips 12, *12, 154,* 156
hairpieces 19
   Fitting and Wearing a False Fringe 81
   Fitting and Wearing a False Ponytail
      82–3
hairspray 17, *17*
hats 150–1, 152, 153
heat-protective sprays 17
heated appliances 14–15
heated rollers *13,* 15, *15,* 64
hot brushes 15
hot sticks 15, *15*

irons
   crimping 15
   straightening *14,* 15
   Using Irons to Create Flicks in Layered
      or Graduated Hair 55
   Using Irons to Create Movement
      in Longer Hair 58–9
   Using Irons to Create Movement
      in Shorter Hair 54
   Using Irons to Create Striking Blades
      in Shorter Hair 52–3
   Using Irons to Straighten Hair for a
      Super-sleek Look 56–7

longer hair
   Blow-drying Longer Hair for a Smooth
      Finish 40–1

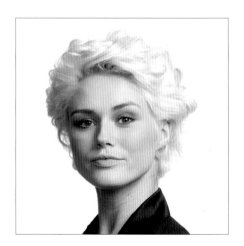

Blow-drying Longer Hair for Volume and Movement 42–3
Blow-drying Mid-length or Longer Hair for a Loose Finish 37
Creating a Rolling Ponytail on Mid-length or Longer Hair 86–7
Creating a Textured Twist Up-do on Longer Hair 102–3
Creating a Twist Up-do on Longer Hair 127
Using Irons to Create Movement in Longer Hair 58–9
Using Mousse to Create a Bedhead Finish on Longer Hair 76

Marcel waves 72, *see also* waves
mid-length hair
Blow-drying Mid-length Hair for a Bedhead Finish 39
Blow-drying Mid-length Hair for a Soft, Relaxed Look 28–9
Blow-drying Fringed Mid-Length Hair for a Textured Finish 36
Blow-drying Mid-length Hair for All-over Texture 35
Blow-drying Mid-length or Longer Hair for a Loose Finish 37
Creating a Mussed-up Back-do on Mid-length Hair 128–9
Creating a Pin-up on Mid-length Hair 124–5
Creating a Quick Party Look on Mid-length Hair 110–11
Creating a Rolling Ponytail on Mid-length or Longer Hair 86–7
Creating a Twist Back-do on Mid-length Hair 126
mousse 18, 76

party look
Creating a Quick, Chic Party Look on Shorter Hair 108–9
Creating a Quick Party Look on Curly Hair 112–13
Creating a Quick Party Look on Mid-length Hair 110–11
pin curls
Using Pin Curls to Create a Gentle, Tumbling Curl 68
pin-ups
Creating a Glamorous Pin-up on Shorter Curly Hair 107

Creating a Pin-up on Mid-length Hair 124–5
Creating a Romantic Wedding Pin-up 148
plaits 19
Creating a Perfect Plaited Ponytail 90–1
Using Multi-plaits to Create a Stronger Wave 71
Using Plaits to Create a Gentle Wave 70
polishes 17
pomades 17
ponytails
Creating a Perfect Plaited Ponytail 90–1
Creating a Rolling Ponytail on Mid-length or Longer Hair 86–7
Creating Sophisticated Ponytails for Special Events 118–19
Fitting and Wearing a False Ponytail 82–3
Placing Ponytails for Different Effects 88–9

rag-rolling hair 13
ribbons 154, 157
rollers 13, *13*, *18*
heated *13*, 15, *15*
Setting Hair on Heated Rollers 64
Setting Hair on Self-gripping Rollers 65

scrunch drying 18
self-gripping rollers
Setting Hair on Self-Gripping Rollers 65
serums 17
setting techniques 18–19
shine sprays 17
shorter hair
Blow-drying Shorter Hair for a Chic, Grown-up Look 24
Blow-drying Shorter Hair for a Multi-texture Effect 30–1
Blow-drying Shorter Hair for a Sleek, Shiny Finish 25
Blow-drying Shorter Hair for a Smooth Finish 22
Blow-drying Shorter Hair for a Soft, Relaxed Look 28–9
Blow-drying Shorter Hair for a Textured Finish 32
Blow-drying Shorter Hair Smooth with Kicked-out Ends 23
Blow-drying to Add Contrast to a Shorter Textured Style 33

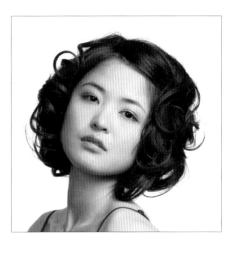

Blow-drying to Add Volume and Choppy Texture to Shorter Hair 34
Creating a Glamorous Pin-up on Shorter Curly Hair 107
Creating a Quick, Chic Party Look on Shorter Hair 108–9
Tonging Shorter Hair for Texture 47
Using Gel to Create a Smooth, Wet Look on Shorter Hair 74
Using Gel to Create Spikes on Shorter Hair 75
Using Irons to Create Movement in Shorter Hair 54
Using Irons to Create Striking Blades in Shorter Hair 52–3
Using Your Fingers to Shape Shorter Hair 73
sleek finish
Blow-drying Shorter Hair for a Sleek, Shiny Finish 25
Creating a Sleek, Elegant Finish on Shorter Hair 106
smooth look
Blow-drying Curly Hair for a Soft, Smooth Look 44–5
Blow-drying Longer Hair for a Smooth Finish 40–1
Blow-drying Shorter Hair for a Chic, Grown-up Look 24
spikes
Using Gel to Create Spikes on Shorter Hair 75
straight hair
Creating Sumptuous Curls on Straight Hair 116–17
Using Irons to Straighten Hair for a Super-sleek Look 56–7
styling products 16–17

styling tools 10–11
  combs 12, *12*
  hairbrushes 10–11, *10, 11*
  pins and clips 12, *12*
  rollers 13, *13*
  shapers or rods 13, *13*

tiaras 154
tonging
  Creating a Chic, Tonged
    Tumbling Up-do 138–9
  Tonging Shorter Hair for Texture 47
  Using Tongs for Different Curled
    Effects 48–9
  Using Tongs to Create Random Spiral
    Curls 50
tongs *14*, 15

up-dos
  Creating a Chic, Tonged Tumbling
    Up-do 138–9

Creating a Chic Wedding Up-do 149
Creating a Textured Twist Up-do on
  Longer Hair 102–3
Creating a Twist Up-do on Longer Hair
  127
Creating an Elegant Top Roll Up-do
  134–5
Creating an Up-do on Crimped Hair
  142–3
Creating an Up-do on Curly Hair 140–1
Creating an Up-do with a Front Roll
  Detail 136–7

vertical rolls 19

waves
  Creating a Perfect Wave Set 114–15
  Using Irons to Create Movement
    in Longer Hair 58–9
  Using Multi-plaits to Create a Stronger
    Wave 71

Using Plaits to Create a Gentle
  Wave 70
  see also Marcel wave
weddings
  Creating a Chic Wedding Up-do
    149
  Creating a Classic Wedding Back-do
    147
  Creating a Contemporary Wedding
    Back-do 146
  Creating a Loose Wedding Style 144
  Creating a Romantic Wedding
    Pin-up 148
  Creating a Stylish Wedding
    Back-do 145
Wearing a Hat 150–1
wigs 19
  Fitting and Wearing a Whole-head
    Wig 78–9
  Fitting and Wearing a Wig with a
    Natural Hair Fringe 77

Acknowledgements

Thank you to Goldwell & KMS California for supplying styling products and arranging their partner hairdressers and for the use of The Goldwell Academy in Mayfair. Particular thanks for help and support to:
• William Wilson – Head of Creative Direction (Goldwell & KMS)
• Sarah Clohessy – Marketing Director (Goldwell & KMS)
• Samantha Field – PR & Marketing (Goldwell & KMS)

The Publisher and Nicky Pope would also like to thank the following for their hard work during the photoshoots or for supplying equipment:

Hairdressing team
• Mo Nabbach at M&M Hair Academy, London
• Margaret Nabbach at M&M Hair Academy, London
• Rachel Hurley, Educator at The Goldwell Academy, London
• Kelly Stone at Elements, Bishops Stortford

• Michael Barnes at Michael Barnes Hairdressing, Covent Garden
• Amanda Brooke at Hair Associates, Taunton
• Claire Cole at Hair Associates, Kingston-upon-Thames
• Angie Mitchell at Desmond Murray Hairdressing, Covent Garden
• Ross Dilanda at Scully Scully, Godalming

Styling
• Clothes supplied and models dressed by Bernard Connolly, clothes stylist

Make-up
• Tracey Wilmot
• Liz Arimoro
• Linda Andersson

Hair appliances and tools
• All hair appliances and some tools and equipment supplied by BaByliss Pro (www.babyliss.co.uk)

Accessories
• Hair extensions by American Dream (www.americandreamextensions.com)

• Hair ornaments and accessories supplied by Johnny Loves Rosie (www.johnnylovesrosie.co.uk)

Hats and headpieces
• Philip Somerville
• Philip Treacy
• Chanel
• Dior

Picture Credits
All pictures © Anness Publishing Ltd, apart from the following:
t = top; b = bottom; r = right; l = left; c = centre
Babyliss 10, 11, 12bc, 13tl, 14, 15.
Corbis 11tl (Rich Gomez/Corbis).
iStockphoto 6 (Quavondo Nguyen), 10 tr (S. Hogge), 12bl (N. Siverina), 12br (C. Baldini), 12tc (A. Balcazar), 12tr, 13tc (V. Anyakin), 13bl (L. Gagne), 13br (E. Bonzami), 16, 17t (K. Deprey), 17b, 18bl, 18tr, 19 (L. Williams), 152 (1), 152 (2) (S. Radosavljevic), 152 (3) (P. Han), 152 (4) (P. Hakimata), 154bl, 154bc (T. England), 154tc (J. Fontanella), 154tcr (M. Baysan), 157 (2) (A. Bryukhanova).
Johnny Loves Rosie 154ct, 154tr.